ophthalmic imaging

For Elsevier:

Commissioning Editor: Robert Edwards
Development Editor: Veronika Watkins
Project Manager: Emma Riley
Designer: George Ajayi
Illustration Manager: Merlyn Harvey
Illustrator: Precision Illustration

eye essentials

ophthalmic imaging

James S. Wolffsohn PhD PgC PgDipAdvClinOptom
Professor, School of Life and Health Sciences, Aston University, UK

SERIES EDITORS
Sandip Doshi PhD MCOptom
Optometrist in private practice, Hove East Sussex, UK
Examiner, College of Optometrists, London, UK
Formerly Clinical Editor, Optician

William Harvey MCOptom
Visiting Clinician and Director of Visual Impairment Clinic, City University, London, UK
Professional Programme Tutor for Boots Opticians Ltd
Clinical Editor, Optician, Reed Business Information, Sutton, UK

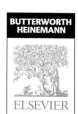

BUTTERWORTH
HEINEMANN

ELSEVIER

EDINBURGH LONDON NEW YORK OXFORD
PHILADELPHIA ST LOUIS SYDNEY TORONTO 2008

BUTTERWORTH
HEINEMANN
ELSEVIER

First published 2008

ISBN: 978-0-7506-8857-4

British Library Cataloguing in Publication Data
A catalogue record for this book is available from the British Library

Library of Congress Cataloging in Publication Data
A catalog record for this book is available from the Library of Congress

Notice
Neither the Publisher nor the Author assume any responsibility for any loss or injury and/or damage to persons or property arising out of or related to any use of the material contained in this book. It is the responsibility of the treating practitioner, relying on independent expertise and knowledge of the patient, to determine the best treatment and method of application for the patient.

The Publisher

Printed in China

Dedicated to my ever supportive family, in particular my wife Rachel and son Peter

Contents

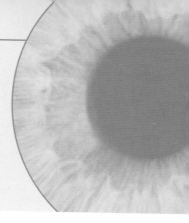

Foreword

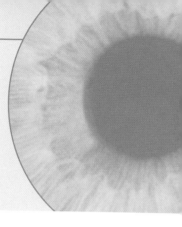

Eye Essentials is a series of books intended to cover the core skills required by the eye care practitioner in general and/or specialized practice. It consists of books covering a wide range of topics, ranging from: routine eye examination to assessment and management of low vision; assessment and investigative techniques to digital imaging; case reports and law to contact lenses.

Authors known for their interest and expertise in their particular subject have contributed books to this series. The reader will know many of them, as they have published widely within their respective fields. Each author has addressed key topics in their subject in a practical rather than theoretical approach, hence each book has a particular relevance to everyday practice.

Each book in the series follows a similar format and has been designed to enable the reader to ascertain information easily and quickly. Each chapter has been produced in a user-friendly format, thus providing the reader with a rapid-reference book that is easy to use in the consulting room or in the practitioner's free time.

Optometry and dispensing optics are continually developing professions, with the emphasis in each being redefined as we learn more from research and as technology stamps its mark. The *Eye Essentials* series is particularly relevant to the practitioner's requirements and as such will appeal to students,

x

graduates sitting professional examinations and qualified practitioners alike. We hope you enjoy reading these books as much as we have enjoyed producing them.

Sandip Doshi
Bill Harvey

Preface

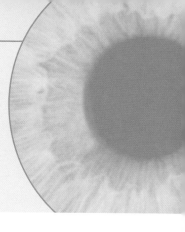

Enhanced imaging is one of the most exciting developments in healthcare of the eyes. It enables a better understanding of the differences between individuals (physiological variation) and how this may affect choices in laser refractive surgery and intraocular lens choice, for example. Perhaps more importantly, it allows the detection of changes in the structure of the eye, such as in the macular region, improving the ability to detect disease, to establish the best treatment strategy, and to monitor the subsequent changes that occur. The technology is already reaching the level of photoreceptor resolution which will help in our understanding of eye disease and enable new treatments to be developed. Further advances in imaging may allow us to better understand the individual's ocular physiology rather than just anatomical structure.

Ocular imaging is a rapidly advancing field and some of the technology explained in this book will be superseded in a short period of time. However, the book purposely explains and demonstrates the complete technology involved with imaging, from imaging chip and colour information capture to high-end instrumentation as this is critical to a full understanding of the potential and limitations of ocular imaging. I hope you find this book as interesting and enjoyable as I have in writing it.

James Wolffsohn

Acknowledgements

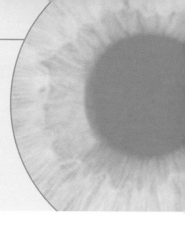

The author gratefully acknowledges Rachael Peterson for her support, data collection and superb images. Also collaborative work with Clare O'Donnell on corneal transparency, Christine Purslow with digital imaging, Peter Hurcomb with imaging in systemic hypertension, Leon Davies and Shehzad Naroo with anterior eye imaging, and Krish Singh and Hannah Bartlett on MRI.

Clinical and Experimental Optometry kindly allowed use of some material in the anterior eye imaging chapter (Chapter 4) which has previously been published (Wolffsohn J S, Peterson R C (2006) Anterior ophthalmic imaging. *Clinical and Experimental Optometry* 89:205–214). Jon Gibson kindly provided the figure on angiography in Chapter 5 (Fig. 5.6).

The author does not have any commercial or proprietary interest in any of the techniques mentioned in this review.

1
Importance of ophthalmic imaging

Computer imaging is becoming more common in our everyday lives. Whether it is having your holiday snaps on CD, digital cameras, e-mail attachments or work presentations, the advantages of electronic imaging and storage are attracting much attention and usage. Not surprisingly, ophthalmic documentation is not far behind. Medical and allied professions have always emphasized the need for recording what clinicians have observed, but the time needed to sketch interesting features and the accuracy of the finished result have not been ideal. The use of film-based photography in optometric documentation has long been advocated as a better alternative, but it is expensive and the delay between taking the photographs and observing the results makes poor images difficult to replace and rapid monitoring awkward to achieve (Cox 1995). Computer imaging (often referred to as 'digital imagery') can offer increased flexibility and improved storage, comparison facilities, image enhancement and analysis.

However, the use of imaging in ophthalmic practice goes beyond just recording what clinicians have observed. For example, imaging sensors are used in videotopographers, some autorefractors, aberrometers, visual field analysers (for eye fixation monitoring) and low-vision electronic vision enhancement systems (often referred to as closed-circuit televisions). Other technologies such as scanning laser ophthalmoscopy, confocal microscopy, magnetic resonance imaging (MRI) and ultrasonography can also build an image of ocular structures. This book aims to highlight the issues involved with ocular imaging and how such techniques can be best utilized in enhancing ocular diagnosis, monitoring and treatment.

Chapter 2 examines the hardware used in ophthalmic imaging. Imaging chips have developed greatly, particularly with the commercial demand for digital cameras to replace film cameras. This was accelerated by the camera function built into many mobile phones and has resulted in the investment in this technology required for rapid development and a reduction in price. The two main forms of chip are discussed, namely charge-coupled devices (CCDs) and complementary metal oxide semiconductors (CMOS). A newer technology, foveon chips, is also mentioned as a way to achieve 100% spectral and spatial resolution without the expense, light loss and fragility of three-chip cameras. Image transfer from the light capture medium to a computer is one of the main limiting factors to real-time imaging of megapixel images, with 'live' video being of low resolution or jerky. Knowledge of digital image interfaces is of interest not just to video capture, but also to the ability to capture optimized static images of the ocular surfaces. Much emphasis is placed on camera resolution, but higher resolution requires larger and more efficient storage options. Optical and lighting hardware considerations are often overlooked when purchasing imaging devices in favour of camera characteristics, but are critical for optimal imaging. Image illumination is controlled by shutter speed (at the expense of image blur for fast moving objects) and aperture size (at the expense of depth of focus). Flash units can overcome these disadvantages, but make the captured image less predictable. Finally, no matter how good your captured image, if a hard copy is required printing issues need to be considered.

Once an image has been captured, it needs to be stored and manipulated. Imaging software is discussed in Chapter 3. Software also has an increasingly important role in controlling imaging hardware, allowing more user-friendly and 'intelligent' user interfaces. Because of the commercial availability of cameras, beam splitters and slit-lamp biomicroscopes, many attempts have been made to design simple imaging solutions, but they often fail due to a poor interface with computer software. Easy access to the images of a patient, following progression, objective grading, image analysing, enhancing and labelling are all essential to good ophthalmic imaging. Image compression algorithms are widely used to make complex images more usable, but care must be taken not to compromise the quality of the image captured. With improvements in image technology, more importance has been placed on the capture and editing of movies to allow more realistic presentation of techniques, ocular devices and ocular conditions.

For ophthalmic imaging, considerations can be neatly broken down into anterior eye and posterior eye regions. Few instruments can image both regions, without major changes in hardware, although more general instrumentation is attracting much interest. The slit-lamp biomicroscope is a key and diverse instrument in eye care. Beam splitters have long been integrated to split the eye-piece view to a second observer or image capture device. Newer systems have integrated the camera into the body of the slit-lamp to produce a more compact, stylish device than many bolt-on systems. Illumination techniques and their uses are reviewed in Chapter 4, along with the imaging of the essential vital dye, fluorescein. Other anterior eye imaging techniques include: corneal topography, to assess the curvature of the corneal surfaces through reflection or scanning slit techniques; confocal microscopy, to produce high resolution images of the corneal structure; optical coherence tomography, a well-established macular assessment technique which has now been applied to anterior segment imaging; ultrasonography, previously the main technique for assessing corneal and crystalline lens thickness, but now being used more when light-based non-invasive techniques fail; and more expensive body imaging techniques such as computerized tomography and magnetic resonance imaging.

Posterior eye imaging is covered in Chapter 5. Fundus cameras are becoming more commonplace in eye care practice, with systems allowing advanced imaging techniques such as 'stitching' of mosaic composites and stereoscopic viewing. Hardware and software considerations discussed in Chapters 2 and 3 are important to the optimization of image capture. Newer instruments combine basic fundus imaging with visual field light sensitivity information (retinal microperimeter) and achieve a wider field of view and reduced light scatter with scanning techniques (scanning laser ophthalmoscopes, optical coherence tomography and scanning laser polarimetry). Other techniques such as ultrasonography, computerized tomography and magnetic resonance imaging take advantage of non-light techniques to penetrate deeper into the eye and avoid optical distortion effects.

The imaging considerations of different surfaces of the eye are considered in Chapter 6. This provides clinicians with different options to consider when changes are suspected or detected, to improve diagnosis and monitoring of the condition. Finally Chapter 7 is dedicated to the evolving area of telemedicine, where the limitations of geographical location are minimized by the transmission of images to allow quicker and more expert interpretations of changes, to improve treatment of complex conditions.

Whether you are in an ophthalmic clinical practice, research or manufacture, you cannot ignore the advances in ophthalmic imaging. Few advanced instruments do not involve some element of imaging. Living in a more litigious society demands that proof is available regarding past reality. Imaging offers us improved visualization and grading of conditions, and the ability to refer to the past without relying on having seen the patient on previous visits, or on intensive record keeping or a fantastic memory. Even if we don't have the instrumentation ourselves, knowledge of what new techniques are capable of and which are appropriate, as well as being able to communicate what the patient will experience are critical. So with the falling cost of basic ophthalmic imaging devices, can you afford to remain ignorant?

2
Hardware

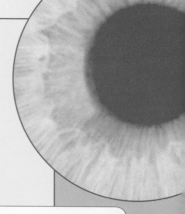

Whenever one mentions an electronic imaging system, resolution seems to be the key feature that is emphasized. However, a full understanding of the mechanism of imaging technology and the optical system as a whole is necessary to optimize ocular imaging.

Light capture medium

A traditional analogue camera is a basic device, exposing a piece of film through a lens and shutter. Photographic films are coated with crystals of a silver halide, usually silver bromide. The crystal atoms are electrically charged, with positively charged silver ions and negatively charged bromide ions. These are maintained in an evenly spaced cubic grid by their electrical attraction. When the film is exposed to light energy, the photons of light release electrons from bromide ions, which collect at defects in the crystal (sensitivity specks), which in turn attract an equal number of free silver ions. The combination is silver atoms (black deposits), which in the processing stage are amplified by chemicals to a negative image.

Usually 24 or 36 images are recorded on one film and processing takes some time, interrupting the continuity of care of a patient and adding to administration of patient files, and whether the images were good enough quality cannot be assessed immediately with the patient present. Polaroid™ film had the advantage of almost instant development, but the image quality and durability was inferior to 35 mm colour transparencies. The complexity is in the design of the film and the processing stage. In comparison, digital cameras are more complex, with the image processing undertaken internally by the cameras' electronics. Few 'digital' photo-sensors are as large as a piece of 35 mm film, so camera lenses have to be longer (typically 1.4–1.6×). Digital images can be viewed instantaneously on a monitor, enhanced or magnified and stored on a computer or memory stick. It should also be noted that if dirt or dust enters a camera on changing a lens or fitting to an optical system, whereas for a film camera this normally only damages a single picture, with a digital camera it will continue to affect images until it is removed.

Digital images are a made up of a matrix of light intensity points called pixels (picture elements). Digital cameras typically have one of three types of light detection chip (Fig. 2.1):

1. **CCD** (charge-coupled device – a description of the technology used to move and store the electron charge). CCDs consist of etched pixelated metal oxide semiconductors made from silicon, sensitive in the visible and near infrared spectrum. They convert light that falls onto them into electrons, sensing the level/amount of light rather than colour. Only the photon-to-electron conversion is conducted on the pixel, allowing the maximum amount of space to remain within each pixel for capturing light information. They therefore have a low signal-to-noise ratio. The electron-to-voltage conversion is done on the chip, leaving the supporting camera circuitry (three to eight additional chips) to digitize this analogue data.

2. **CMOS** (complementary metal oxide semiconductor – technology used to make a transistor on a silicon wafer). CMOS chips are similar to CCDs, but both the photon-to-electron and electron-to-voltage conversion are conducted within the pixel together with digitization of the signal, leaving less room for the light-sensitive part of the sensor. Normally a microlens is used to capture more light within the pixel area and bend it towards the light-sensitive part (the fill factor) of the pixel. CMOS have the advantage of being cheaper and less power hungry than CCDs, because they have fewer components, making them more reliable.

3. **Foveon X3** (a chip of transparent quartz containing three layers of CMOS). This newer sensor uses three layers of CMOS imagers embedded in silicon, positioned to take advantage of the fact that silicon absorbs different wavelengths (and hence colour) of light at different depths. This enables each pixel to record individual and independent values of green, red and blue, providing full and accurate colour data from each pixel.

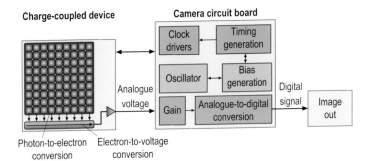

Charge-coupled device

Camera circuit board

Analogue voltage

Digital signal

Image out

Photon-to-electron conversion   Electron-to-voltage conversion

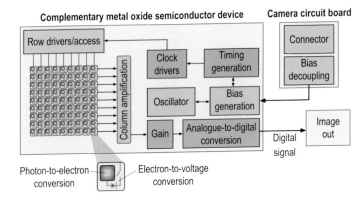

Complementary metal oxide semiconductor device

Camera circuit board

Digital signal

Image out

Photon-to-electron conversion   Electron-to-voltage conversion

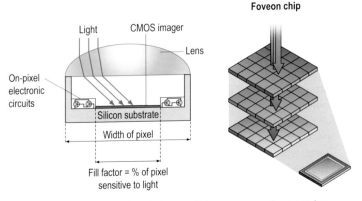

Light   CMOS imager

Lens

On-pixel electronic circuits

Silicon substrate

Width of pixel

Fill factor = % of pixel sensitive to light

Foveon chip

Figure 2.1 CCD, CMOS and Foveon light capture and processing (reproduced with permission from TASi).

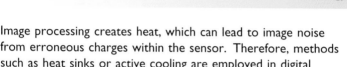

Image processing creates heat, which can lead to image noise from erroneous charges within the sensor. Therefore, methods such as heat sinks or active cooling are employed in digital cameras. In an over-humid environment, over-cooling can lead to condensation causing chip damage. As noted previously, CMOS technology is less power-demanding than CCDs and therefore requires less cooling. Although most pixels are square or rectangular, more hexagonal style designs are being created to allow tighter arrangement and hence more efficient imagers.

Capture technology

Most optometric imaging needs the versatility of capturing both dynamic and static objects and therefore uses a matrix or grid of CCD/CMOS elements (area array). Progressive scanning cameras (such as those used in flatbed scanners) do exist, with a sensor consisting of three parallel lines of CCD pixels (coated with red, green or blue filters) that are gradually moved across an image by a stepper motor and lead screw, building up a complete colour image with accurate colour data at every pixel position. However, exposure times are long, requiring continuous light and a very stable image. Area array imaging only allows each pixel to capture one colour in a single exposure (shot; Fig. 2.2), so to create full colour information the camera can be:

1. **Single matrix, one shot** – each pixel coated in a different colour, spatially arranged in a mosaic pattern (providing twice as many green as red or blue pixels, based upon the Bayer pattern; Fig. 2.2). The image is then processed (interpolation of colour data from the surrounding pixels) to an image with the full resolution of the chip, with 100% spatial, but only 90–95% spectral fidelity. This can result in colour fringing around sharp edges, although more modern interpolation algorithms have reduced this effect. Interpolation requires a significant amount of processing, which takes both time and power to accomplish (Fig. 2.3a).

2. **Single matrix, three shot** – instead of individually coating pixels, three shots are taken through a red, green and blue

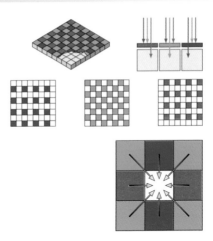

Figure 2.2 Single-chip, one-shot cameras use an area array matrix of red, green and blue typically based upon the Bayer pattern. The colour of each pixel location is established from a balance of the intensity of light passing through its colour filter and the colour of all the surrounding pixels (reproduced with permission from TASi).

filter in succession, allowing each pixel to collect full data for that individual pixel position. Although there are three separate exposures, capture time is fast due to no processor intensive interpolation (Fig. 2.3b).

3. **Single matrix, one/three shot** – this works as a single-matrix, one-shot camera for action shots, but for static imagery can be switched so that the pixel matrix is shifted by one pixel between shots to allow the same pixel position to take consecutive readings in red, green and blue (Fig. 2.3c).

4. **Single matrix, macroshift** – the limitation for all area array cameras is the physical pixel dimensions of currently available CCD and CMOS sensors, so these cameras take multiple exposures, moving the sensor between shots, and use 'stitching' software to create the final image. They work best for stationary, constantly lit targets and have a relatively slow capture process (Fig. 2.3d).

5. **Triple matrix, one shot (often called three-chip cameras)** – each chip captures an image of the scene at its

Single matrix – one shot

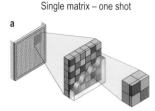

a

Single matrix – macroshift

d

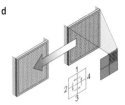

Single matrix – three shot

b

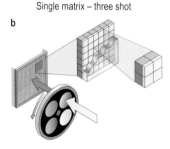

Triple matrix – one shot

e

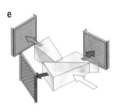

Single matrix – one/three shot

c

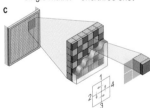

Figure 2.3 Principle of: **(a)** single-chip, one-shot camera; **(b)** single-chip, three-shot camera; **(c)** single-chip, one/three-shot camera; **(d)** single-chip, macroshift camera; **(e)** three-chip, one-shot camera (reproduced with permission from TASi).

full resolution, but through a different filter (red, green or blue). Prisms behind the lens aperture allow green filtered light to pass undiverted to their chip, whereas red and blue light is diverted to their respective chips on either side of the 'green' chip. The processing converts the image to the

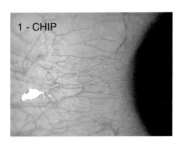
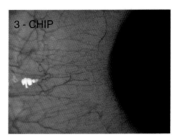

Figure 2.4 Comparison of a resolution-matched image from a three-chip (right) and single-chip (left) camera taken through the same slit-lamp optics. Notice the similar coloration between the two images, but the reduced luminance of the image from the three-chip camera.

resolution of one chip (not the resolution of one chip times three as is sometimes suggested) with absolute data for red, green and blue light allowing 100% spatial and spectral fidelity. These cameras are more expensive, delicate, heavy and bulky than single-matrix cameras and due to the light loss from the two beam splitters, require a higher light output from the slit-lamp for equivalent performance (Figs 2.3e; 2.4).

The physical action necessary to capture an image differs between systems, with more purpose-built systems favouring a joystick button or foot-pedal, in addition to software or camera control.

Image transfer

A delay between capturing an image and being able to capture another can be frustrating in a dynamic capture situation. Image transfer from the camera hardware to the computer for storage or manipulation can be divided into analogue and digital formats.

Analogue transfer

Analogue transfer involves sending a composite stream of voltage values (relating to image position intensity) and a timed pulse created by the imager, through a BNC (bayonet Neill–Concelman) or phono connector on the rear of the camera. This suffers from system noise interpreted as a change in intensity and timing errors interpreted as a change in localization. S-video is a two-wire system and as such is a more robust format, with chroma (colour) and luminance (greyscale intensity) information transmitted separately. High-end analogue systems transmit red, green and blue signals on separate data lines and a synchronizing pulse on the fourth wire. Therefore the signal-to-noise ratio is lower, but the computer board required to input the data and reassemble it into an image is more expensive than simpler analogue formats. It is important to note that although many cameras are described as 'digital' because they use a CCD/CMOS for capturing the photons of light, for simplicity and cheapness they use a composite output (such as a BNC) connector to transmit the image and analogue image capture cards, losing some of the benefits of the digital image capture.

Digital transfer

Digital transfer sends a signal in bytes ('0's or '1's) and so noise to the system is unlikely to affect the image. For example, signal noise of +0.05 V would convert an intensity of 0.52 V on a 0.00–1.00 V range to 0.57 V, indicating a different intensity to that measured, reducing colour and luminance fidelity, whereas this would not be enough to alter the byte value over the same voltage range (as 0.05 V would still be translated as 0.00 V by the image processing). Obviously a great deal more data is processed and so the connector to the computer has multiple pins. This type of interface can cope with 'megapixel' images (usually referring to images with more than a million pixels, approximately twice the resolution of the typical 768×568 PAL image – see p. 17). However, transfer speed is often limited to below the 25 Hz (PAL/SECAM) or 30 Hz (NTSC) interlaced image transfer speed of analogue. The average critical flicker fusion frequency of the human eye is typically between 35 and 50 Hz and so any image frames presented for greater than 30 ms should appear as a smooth image (Lachenmayr et al 1994). Higher resolution digital images create so much data that even at the fastest transfer speed, the image can only be transferred and displayed at <20 Hz and the video image appears jerky. However, although a higher frame rate allows a smooth, continuous real-time image, the greater the presentation frequency of the camera, the less the potential exposure time of the pixel receptors to light, leading to a lower (worse) signal-to-noise ratio.

There are a number of interfaces that are currently used to connect digital cameras or card readers direct to a computer:

1. **Small computer system interface (SCSI)** – used more often with high-end scanners than digital cameras, offers a reasonable transfer speed (Ultra 2 SCSI transfers data at a rate of 40 MB/s), but is limited to a short cable length and is generally difficult to set up (needing to be turned on before the host computer and with each device needing a unique identifying number).
2. **Universal serial bus (USB)** – allows autoconfiguration and plug-and-play technology, also providing a small external power source (500 mA). The slow transfer speed of USB1 (1.5 MB/s) has been improved with USB2 (up to 60 MB/s).
3. **FireWire** – a high speed serial bus defined by IEEE standard 1394 which provides autoconfiguration and plug-and-play technology. It is robust and easy to use, allowing transfer speeds of ≥50 MB/s. The interface also allows the hardware (in this case the camera) to be controlled from the software, such as altering the shutter speed, iris diameter and image gain (light sensitivity). As FireWire was developed specifically for movie transfer, it has a protected bandwidth (memory allocation) so is unaffected by other functions the computer may wish to perform while your movie or image is transferring from your hardware to the computer.

Television video standards

Television video standards dictate how images are created from the captured camera information and differ across the world (Fig. 2.5).

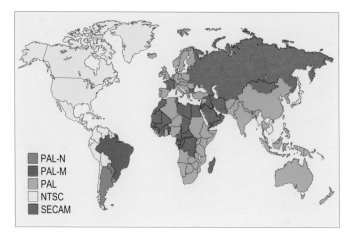

Figure 2.5 Video standards used by different regions of the world.

- **Phase Alternating Line (PAL) video** – the standard for most of Europe and Australasia, and some of Asia and South America. This writes alternate horizontal lines of the screen every 1/50th of a second and interlaces them to a complete image every 1/25th of a second.
- **National Television Standards Committee (NTSC) video** – the North American and Japan standard. It was the first to be introduced in 1953 and writes a smaller number of horizontal lines of the screen (525 versus 625 for PAL), but at a higher rate (1/29.97th of a second).
- **Sequential Couleur Avec Memoire** or **Sequential Colour with Memory (SECAM) video** – introduced in the early 1960s and implemented in France and the former Soviet Union and Eastern bloc countries. It uses the same bandwidth as PAL (also 625 horizontal lines), but transmits the colour information sequentially.

There are also several different versions of each video standard (such as PAL-M and PAL-N – used in South America) which differ in the frequency of their video bandwidth and sound carrier.

Image storage

It is essential to be able to store and access images in ophthalmic practice once they have been captured. Storage can take place 'on-board' the camera in a digital storage media such as CompactFlash, SmartMedia or MicroDrive or by an interface to a tethered computer. Software storage of images will be considered in Chapter 3.

Resolution

Two of the major considerations with digital imaging are the resolution needed to image the object of interest and the compression that can be utilized to minimize the space needed to store the image (Charman 1998). If photographs are to be used to detect pathology, monitor progression and protect against litigation, it is essential that the resolution is sufficient to allow all clinical features of interest to be detected and that this is not compromised by the image storage.

Resolution is the ability to distinguish the difference between two sequential points. In digital imagery, this depends on the number of pixels that the image is composed of (Jensen and Scherfig 1999). Further details of the appropriate camera resolution for anterior eye imaging and fundus imaging are discussed in Chapters 4 and 5, respectively.

Optical considerations

The optics of an imaging system are critical to capturing good images. The quality of any camera image can only be as good as the lens system which captures the light and focuses it on the light receptor. This is even more critical with a matrix camera due to the smaller capture area compared to 35 mm film. The placement of a camera's objective lens in-line with a microscope

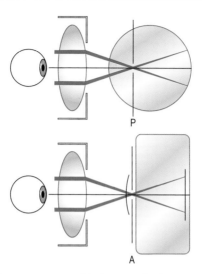

Figure 2.6 Microscope optics (slit-lamp or fundus camera) in conjunction with an eye or digital camera. The pupil is coincident with the camera's aperture and the focal length of the camera is matched to that of the human eye (~60 D).

ocular (slit-lamp or fundus optical body) will only give an in-focus image if the camera optics equals the power of the observer eye (Fig. 2.6). Therefore the focal length of the camera's optical system needs to be approximately 17 mm (= 1/60 D; Schirmer 2004). Features such as the type of zoom (continuous or fixed level) should also be considered.

As well as the type of light receptor chip used (e.g. CCD or CMOS), the size of chip should also be noted (normally ¼ to ¾ of an inch). Each pixel receptor will obviously be larger on a larger chip of the same resolution as a smaller chip. The bigger the pixel receptor target, the more chance the photon has of hitting it. The latest digital cameras, boasting resolutions of greater than 6 million pixels on a ½ inch chip, have pixel receptors of <1 µm in diameter and therefore are limited by the size of a photon. The image looks good and takes up plenty of disk size, but when magnified can appear blurred.

Lighting considerations

Appropriate lighting is essential to taking a clear, detailed image. If there is too little light, it is harder to focus the image and detail is difficult to resolve. However, too much lighting can also decrease clarity due to bleaching and light scatter, not forgetting the unnecessary discomfort caused to the patient.

Shutter speed

Shutter speed is controlled mechanically in analogue cameras to physically expose the film to light for a predetermined period of time. Digital cameras have the advantage of being able to 'turn on' the light receptor for a set period of time (electronic shutter), which involves no moving parts. Although this can always be controlled from the camera body, more advanced systems allow shutter speed to be directly controlled from the software. Preset settings can then be programmed to optimize particular images such as corneal transparency and fluorescein imaging. A slower (longer) shutter speed allows a longer period for light to be integrated (hence a higher exposed image), but any movement of the image during this period will lead to blur (Fig. 2.7).

Aperture size

Aperture size can be used in some camera systems to alter the luminance of the image. The aperture controls the intensity of light reaching the imaging chip, in comparison to the shutter speed, which determines the period over which the light intensity is integrated (Fig. 2.8). Aperture size is normally defined as the f-numbers (also known as stops). The f-numbers follow an internationally agreed sequence relating to brightness of the image, with each change to the next highest number halving the amount of light passing to the imaging chip. The f-number denotes the number of times the effective diameter of the aperture divides into the focal length. Therefore it takes into

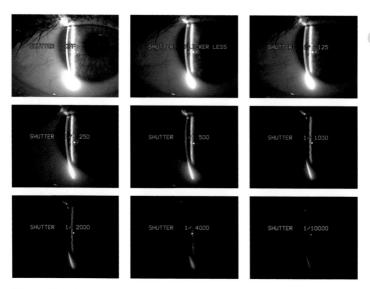

Figure 2.7 An optical section taken with a range of shutter speeds using a slit-lamp biomicroscope.

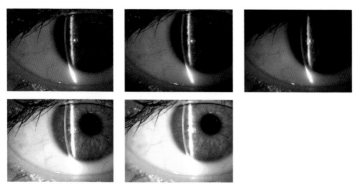

Figure 2.8 An optical section taken with a range of aperture sizes. Top left: minimum aperture. Top middle: ¼ open. Top right: ½ open. Bottom left: ¾ open. Bottom right: fully open.

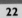
account the two main factors that control how bright an image is formed as:

$$\text{Image brightness} \propto \frac{\text{light intensity}}{\text{distance}^2}$$

Light intensity will increase as the square of the diameter of the lens aperture. Doubling the diameter of the aperture will increase its area (and hence light intensity) by four times.

The depth of focus of the system is reduced when the aperture size is increased. However, if the aperture is decreased too much, diffraction effects start to disrupt the image. The upper limit of the aperture size is usually dependent on the cost effectiveness of a minimal aberration lens. However, wider apertures allow more light to pass through in the same time shutter interval, making the camera more light efficient.

Additional lighting

Additional lighting is essential for ophthalmic imaging due to the loss of light from intervening beam splitters and lenses, incomplete fill factor of the sensor pixels and a reduced light sensitivity compared to the human eye. This is particularly the case for blue/ultraviolet illumination. CCD and CMOS photoreceptors are more responsive to the red end of the spectrum. Therefore they often have an infrared filter in the light path and compensate for the low blue sensitivity by amplifying blue signals within the image processing. Therefore, the blue channel is likely to exhibit more noise than the red or green channels and can be a good way to examine the quality of a digital camera (TASi 2003). Cameras which have low light sensitivity are particularly beneficial for ocular imaging as they allow lower light levels to be used, making the patient more comfortable and the pupils to remain larger. Unfortunately some manufacturers define light sensitivity in terms of lux and others in terms of an emulsion speed figure such as the International Organization for Standardization (ISO) format. The latter was the conventional way of defining film sensitivity to light, with higher ISO films (such as ISO 400/27° or greater) requiring less light in order to give adequate picture exposure in low light conditions, but result in a more coarse appearance to the image. The first ISO figure doubles with each doubling of light sensitivity. The second number marked with a degree sign, often not quoted, increases by 3 with each doubling of sensitivity.

Additional lighting originates from one of three sources:

1. **Internal slit-lamp light unit** can have a fibreoptic attachment diverting some additional illumination towards the front of the eye. The intensity can be controlled by apertures along the fibreoptic light path. However, the rheostat controlling the slit-lamp light unit will also affect the intensity. The head of the fibreoptic attachment is usually positioned to reflect off the illumination system mirror into the eye, giving a diffuse illumination across the whole field of view of the slit-lamp image. As the light path does not follow the traditional slit-lamp illumination path with its intervening apertures and filters, this form of lighting is of limited value in enhancing fluorescein images for example (Fig. 2.9).

2. **External source** can be used to illuminate the eye in a similar way to the fibreoptic attachment. An additional power supply for the lamp unit is usually required. This light source is independent of the slit-lamp's light source and will have a rheostat to control its intensity. Ideally it should have an option to insert a blue filter into its light path for fluorescein viewing, but this is often not the case. Commercial desk or

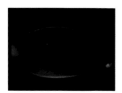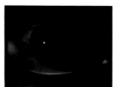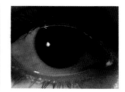

Figure 2.9 Fluorescein viewing with a yellow filter taken with: left: no external illumination; middle: some external white illumination; right: more external white illumination. Note that although the external illumination makes the surrounding eye clearer, the fluorescein dye image is not enhanced.

USB lamps attached to flexible arms can provide a cheap alternative.

3. **Flash** systems are commonly used with retinal imaging and are utilized in some anterior eye cameras. The short flash exposure synchronized with the image capture minimizes the effect of the change in pupil size on the image, but as the resulting image cannot be viewed while setting up the shot, several shots may need to be taken to prevent over- or under-exposure (Figs 2.10 and 2.11). Ideally the flash utilizes

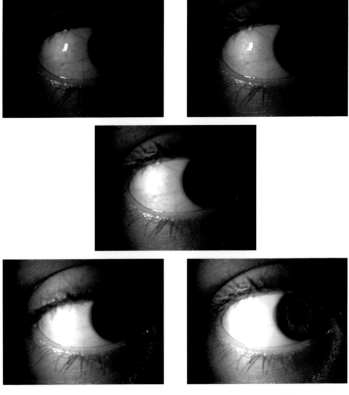

Figure 2.10 An anterior eye image taken with a range of flash intensities. Top left: no flash. Top right: 25% flash. Middle: 50% flash. Bottom left: 75% flash. Bottom right: full flash.

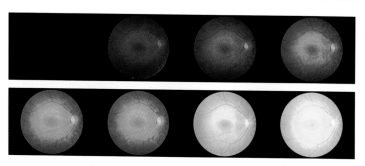

Figure 2.11 A fundus image taken with a range of flash intensities. Increasing flash intensity from top left to bottom right.

the same optical path as the light source used to position the image initially so the visual effect is the same. For example, if you are capturing an optic section of the cornea, the flash should feed into the light path containing the slit aperture, so just the slit of light is enhanced. Hence, if a blue filter is inserted in the light path to view fluorescein staining, using a flash will enhance the image.

Printing

A universal problem encountered when producing colour prints is that monitors and printers are fundamentally different in the way they generate and display images. The ability of a printer to reproduce the colour captured by the camera photo-detector elements is dependent on its colour gamut (also known as colour space). Figure 2.12 displays the colour range of the human eye and the typical gamut of a conventional colour monitor and printer. This shows that both the monitor and printer are a compromise over the human eye, due to the limited subset of pure colours added to black (in the case of monitors) or subtracted from white (in the case of printers) to produce their entire range of hues. Monitors produce all colours by mixing red, green and blue light. Colour printers, on the other hand, typically derive their colour palette by mixing cyan, magenta and yellow

Figure 2.12 Colour range of the human eye compared to typical monitor and printer gamuts. RGB: red, green blue; CMYK: cyan, magenta, yellow, black.

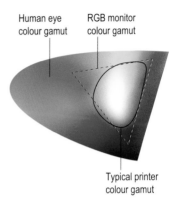

Human eye colour gamut

RGB monitor colour gamut

Typical printer colour gamut

inks with black. Consequently printers cannot produce the vibrant 'pure' reds and greens viewed on monitors.

Despite the fact that perfect colour matching between your monitor and printer is not possible, the colour approximation between the two can be improved by altering the gamma correction of the monitor. Monitors tend to have a non-linear response to brightness levels across their dynamic range (gamma) so most image display programs allow the gamma response to be set. There is an International Colour Consortium (ICC) profile system which if used for the digital camera, monitor and printer will allow as faithful as possible reproduction of colour. Cameras generally have a colour space defined by the International Electrotechnical Commission profile sRGB 61966-2-1, but new higher-end cameras have adopted Adobe RGB colour space with its larger gamut. Unfortunately despite all colour printers having an ICC profile, this is only an approximation as paper absorbs ink to different degrees and the colour of the paper used (such as its whiteness) will affect the resulting image. Using manufacturer specific paper and specifying this correctly in your software will help. However, software can be used to correct for colour inaccuracies between the monitor and printer using a scanner or pre-calibrated colorimeter. It is important to remember that calibration of a monitor only holds for certain lighting conditions. The environmental luminance will affect the perception of colour.

Fade resistance of inkjet printed images is best if they are placed behind glass and not exposed to sunlight. In these circumstances, the best inkjet printed images last as long as 110 years. However, manufacturer's inks and best quality paper need to be used to achieve such fade resistance as they are chemically matched. Generic ink refills fade quickly when exposed to light and generally last less than 1 year.

3
Software

Although imaging systems are often sold on the basis of their hardware features, the software interface with the user is essential to capturing, storing and retrieving the image, all of which have time implications in a busy practice.

Patient image database

Basic, non-optometric specialized software, particularly that available on the retail market for viewing television pictures on your computer, can allow a composite analogue signal to be viewed on a computer and static images to be captured and stored as image files. This software is inexpensive, but does not contain image analysis or patient database facilities. Purpose designed systems not only allow connection to an anterior eye image capture device, but also a fundus camera and a patient management system. Such systems allow a less paper-based practice, and can incorporate a fully integrated patient management, record keeping (including storing images and data capture from all instrumentation) and accountancy package. It is also possible to write and print referral letters and reminder notes from such software. The use of features such as drop-down boxes, 'back'/'undo' buttons and search facilities can reduce the amount of typing and navigation necessary.

It is important for the system to store enough information to be able to locate a patient's data easily (such as surname, forename, date of birth and gender), but not so much compulsory information that it takes ages to prepare for taking an image. All images should automatically be saved under the patient highlighted prior to image capture and preferably under the date of the examination so changes can easily be monitored. Some software requires you to identify where you want to save each image after it has been taken, which can take an age. Others save all images taken for a particular patient in one big block of thumbnails. Thumbnail size and the number that can be viewed at one time is important and ideally should be able to be set to the individual's preferred format (Fig. 3.1). Compression options allow images to be stored at a smaller file size in the database,

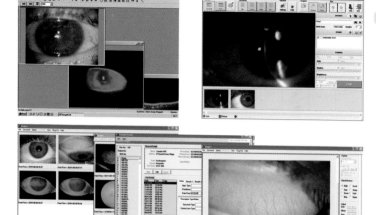

Figure 3.1 A range of different software front-end interfaces.

but you cannot go back to the non-compressed image later if you should need improved resolution (see 'Compression' section on p. 34).

Data stored with the image

As well as storing the image itself, it is important that information relating to the image is also stored. The date and time the image was taken is essential for legal protection. Knowing whether the image taken was from the right or left eye is also important and integrated systems can automatically record this from the position of the instrument optics when the image was captured. The ability to add additional comments about the images is also important and preferably this should be a user-selectable default immediately the image has been taken before the image has been saved. The ability to choose whether the image is saved or not would also be useful as a user-selectable default as sometimes the eyelid disrupts the image or the image does not turn out as planned and if instantly saved, requires subsequent re-entry into the patient image database to delete the image.

Viewing stored images

Once the capture button has been pressed, the user requires to know whether the image captured was what was required or whether a further attempt needs to be made to capture that image. However, as discussed later in the chapter (see 'Movie formats' section on p. 40), a continuous dynamic real-time image is ideal to optimize image capture. Therefore, either the dynamic image can take up only a portion of the monitor screen with the latest image to be captured displayed as a thumbnail image by the side (large enough to see whether the detail required was successfully captured), or the dynamic image can be temporarily frozen showing the captured image (allowing the dynamic and captured image to cover a larger area of the monitor), or a combination of the two methods may be used (Fig. 3.1).

Control of computer hardware

Most camera hardware allow their internal menu options (such as shutter speed and colour setting) to be controlled externally (usually through an RS232 link). This means that this control can be offered to the user through their image capture software to enhance the images they take (see p. 20). This is much easier than trying to master the menu functions of the camera hardware itself and allows predefined settings to be established so that when buttons on the software front panel are clicked on, the camera automatically defaults to the optimum settings for an optical section or fluorescein imaging, for example. The function of the capture button can also be controlled as to whether it captures a static image or a movie. The length of the movie can be preset, or successive clicks of the capture button turn the movie capture on and off.

Importing and exporting images

Sometimes it is necessary to add an image to a patient database, such as from patients' previous notes, and in such cases an import function is necessary. The time and date stamp will indicate when the image was imported, not when the image was taken, and should indicate it to be an imported image. Exporting an image is a more common procedure and allows images to be used for presentations or to be given to a patient, their general medical practitioner or their ophthalmologist. Usually a range of different file format options is available for saving the image, some with a range of quality alternatives on offer. As discussed in the 'Compression' section on page 34, these options should be carefully considered.

Image manipulation

Purpose designed systems usually allow not only the image to be captured, but also for sections of the image to be enlarged, enhanced and annotated (Fig. 3.2). Images can be manipulated in characteristics such as contrast and separating the colour planes (Hom and Bruce 1998). More complex image processing can isolate blood vessels, measure tortuosity and diameter and remove unwanted reflections (Aslam et al 2006). As long as the magnification under which the image was taken is known, the software can allow measurements to be calibrated so, for example, the extension of blood vessels into the cornea can be accurately monitored. Objective grading of ocular characteristics can also be utilized (see 'Objective image analysis' section on p. 67). It is important that the original unannotated image is always available and most systems allow all manipulations to be removed at any time while the image is stored in the database.

Figure 3.2 An annotated anterior eye image.

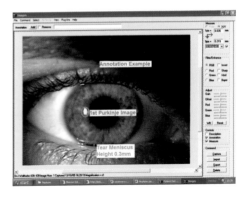

Compatibility

Ideally, the company you purchase your imaging system from also produce the software you will use. However, you may have an existing database you wish to link to or your fundus and anterior eye image capture systems may be from different manufacturers. It is important to check their compatibility and the company's ability to adequately solve any problems that occur or tailor the application to your needs. You may, either now or in the future, want to use the database facility with other computers in the practice and on the front desk, access on-line help facilities or e-mail an image to a colleague for their opinion and therefore networking facilities within the software are necessary. It is also important to consider the availability and cost of support and upgrades to the software as this can prove costly if your version is not supported or you decide to expand your functionality at a later stage.

Compression

Most digital imaging systems offer a selection of different file formats with which to save images and movies. Image compression is a technique to reduce file size, by removing redundant information. In some compression methods the full information can be retrieved (termed 'lossless' formats such as TIFF), but in others the information is permanently deleted ('lossy' formats such as JPEG; Meyler and Burnett Hodd 1998, Garcia et al 2003). There are two main types of graphic formats used to display graphics: vectors and raster (bitmap) files.

Vector files (such as Windows Meta Files [*.wmf] and the 'Pict' format used by Macintosh computers) store images as a series of mathematical descriptions representing simple shapes. The image content is divided into its constituent shapes (such as lines and rectangles), with the file storing their position within the image, shape and colour. The image is then reconstructed from these details when opened. As a result, the image size can be changed without any effect on image quality, but vector files are not really suited to complex images such as real images of the eye. Such images consist of multiple complex shapes with few areas of constant colour.

The whole image of a bitmap graphic file is divided into tiny squares (pixels) and the colour of each pixel recorded. The result is a relatively large file size that cannot be reduced without loss of information. Compression formats aim to reduce the storage space taken up by a file without losing any useful information. Although this works well when the number of colours is limited, it is generally ineffective with continuous tone pictures of high colour depth (such as photographs). Formats include TIFF, RAW, JPEG and BMP.

TIFF (Tagged Image File Format)

This is a lossless format, storing all the data from the camera once its internal processing (such as colour interpolation) has taken place. It uses algorithms to make the file size smaller for storage, but all the compression is reversed on opening. However, the stored images are still relatively large, even larger than the RAW format (see below). For example, a 1600×1200 pixel image in 24-bit colour (3 bytes per pixel) would result in a ~5.8 MB TIFF file.

RAW

RAW is a newer option allowing the captured data to be stored in its raw form, before any processing has taken place. It is relatively simple to calculate the file sizes of RAW images as they consist of 12 bits (or 1.5 bytes) of data per element on the sensor. So for the 1600×1200 pixel sensor described above, a RAW format file of size ~2.9 MB would be created. As discussed, an uncompressed TIFF generated within the camera requires 24 bits for every sensor element so will fill at least twice the storage space of the RAW data. Without a standard, every camera manufacturer records its RAW files differently (although a RAW standard has now been proposed by Adobe). In order to generate a usable image from a RAW file, the same process that the camera would have performed automatically for downloading as a TIFF or JPEG, for example, needs to be conducted by using software on a PC. For example Adobe Photoshop CS comes with a free RAW image format plug-in, which is regularly updated to support new camera models. The main reason for exporting the RAW image is that fine control can be made of colour, tone, sharpness and white balance. The 12-bit dynamic range allows tonal adjustments to be made without the same degree of loss caused when adjusting the levels of an 8-bit dynamic range JPEG or TIFF. Although once any adjustments have been made, the RAW image can be saved in formats such as TIFF or JPEG to share with colleagues, the RAW archived data can always be available for reprocessing.

JPEG (Joint Photographic Experts Group)

This is a compressed format, resulting in the loss of some image integrity. JPEG compression attempts to eliminate redundant or unnecessary information. Red, green and blue (RGB) pixel information is converted into luminance and chrominance components, merging pixels and utilizing compression algorithms (discrete cosine transforms) on 8×8 pixel blocks to remove frequencies not utilized by the human eye (dividing the frequencies by individual quantization coefficient), followed by rounding to integer values. Different compression levels can usually be selected. Using the 1600 × 1200 sensor example, depending on content, a low compression JPEG would be ~0.3 MB. JPEG2000 is the current compression standard introduced in 2001, featuring higher compression, but less image quality loss. Some systems offer a modified JPEG file type known as an Exchangeable Image File (EXIF) which stores 'tags' onto the header of the image file containing technical data such as time, exposure settings and camera make.

BMP (bitmap)

This is Microsoft Windows native bitmap format. Rather than storing each of the red, green and blue (RGB) values necessary for each pixel of a colour image, Microsoft added a customizable palette so that each pixel's colour could then be defined by storing its associated index number rather than the much longer RGB value. This look-up table approach was more efficient for handling images with up to 256 colours as each pixel could be stored in 8 bits of information rather than 24 bits. However, to display 24-bit images, the palette would require over 16 million colours, so each indexed entry would be no smaller than the original RGB value. Therefore the BMP format now stores information as rows or scan lines (i.e. RGBRBGRGB . . .), and the information is compressed by run length encoding (taking repeated sequences and expressing them as number × colour in two bytes).

If all images are stored at maximum quality, archiving can become an issue. Handling large file sizes slows a storage database due to the amount of processing needed, thereby decreasing the advantage of the speed of digital technology. A larger storage area will be needed on the hard drive and back-up medium. Digital images are also easier to distribute such as over the internet if they are relatively small in size (Hom and Bruce 1998).

Several studies have investigated the appropriateness of compression with retinal images. Basu et al (2003) suggested that up to a JPEG compression ratio of 1:20 (between 100% and 75%

JPEG) was appropriate based on objective analysis with lesion counts. Others have identified 75% JPEG as an appropriate limit from subjective analysis of digital images (Newsom et al 2001, Kocsis et al 2003).

Peterson and Wolffsohn (2005) evaluated the most appropriate compression for anterior eye imaging by clinical subjective ranking (20 optometrists) of a range of images (taken by four different cameras) varying in compression (JPEG 100%, 75%, 50%, 25% and 0% quality settings and in BMP format; Fig. 3.3) and by clinical objective grading of the same images

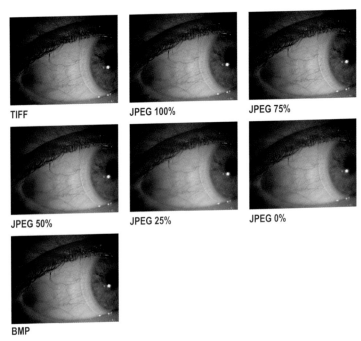

Figure 3.3 An example of the range of compressed images. Note that the difference from the original TIFF image is only just noticeable at JPEG compressions below 50% quality, a reduction in image size of 70×.

(Wolffsohn and Purslow 2003). Up to a 1:70 (50%) JPEG compression could be applied to an image (regardless of the camera which the image was taken on or its pixel resolution) without any apparent loss in subjective image quality. JPEG compression is designed to remove frequencies not utilized by the human eye (by using discrete cosine transforms) and therefore the ability to compress an image by 98.6% (compared to a 2048 × 1360 TIFF) without a loss in subjective image quality confirms that this strategy is successful (Table 3.1). The compression was slightly greater than that suggested as appropriate for retinal images (Newsom et al 2001, Kocsis et al 2003). BMP compression allows an image to be read and displayed more quickly than a TIFF, but as the compression is essentially lossless it is limited in reducing the image size of real images that continuously change in colour tone. BMP compressed images were subjectively rated as of lower image quality than the same resolution TIFF although it is not clear why this was the case. Objective grading of photographs with image analysis (both edge detection and colour extraction) was unaffected even by 0% JPEG compression. It would therefore appear that the frequencies removed by compression do not affect the image parameters examined.

Table 3.1 **Average file size with changes in resolution and image compression and reduction in file size from full resolution TIFF image**

Compression quality	File size (MB)	Reduction (%)
JPEG 100%	848.4	90.2
JPEG 75%	236.0	97.3
JPEG 50%	123.4	98.6
JPEG 25%	79.3	99.1
JPEG 0%	51.9	99.4
BMP	3211.9	62.9

Colour depth

Reducing the number of colours has a significant effect on file size. Each bit of information can either contain a 0 or 1, so 8-bit colour can code $2^8 = 256$ colours (usually greyscales) for each pixel (one byte). High colour (12-bit) can code 65 536 colours and true colour (24-bit) 16 777 216 colour shades (3 bytes per pixel). Less than 24-bit is rarely used to save colour images.

Movie formats

If a picture can speak a thousand words, then the value of a movie file in describing the dynamic nature of anterior eye features (such as blinking and contact lens movement) is virtually invaluable in clinical teaching and presentation. Being able to show a patient their tear film breaking up, or the lack of movement of a contact lens can give strength to the practitioner's suggested management option and enhance their status as a modern health professional.

The role of movie files in retinal imaging may be less obvious, but the ability to review and freeze a momentary view of the fundus when examining a small child or uncooperative patient should not be overlooked. Movies of retinal observation using techniques such as a Volk lens in conjunction with a slit-lamp biomicroscope or a binocular indirect ophthalmoscope can enhance the teaching of the technique, particularly examining the retina whilst viewing the inverted image (so all movements must be diagonally opposite to the direction of fundus one desires to observe). The most common digital video formats are AVI and MPEG.

AVI

AVI (Audio Video Interleave) format was developed by Microsoft, with the initial specification outlined in 1992/3. It is a common format on PCs, and comes with the Windows

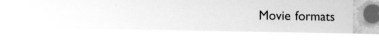
operating system as part of the 'Video for Windows (VfW)' distribution. The format can be *interleaved* (DVEncoder 1) such that video and audio data are stored consecutively in an AVI file (i.e. a segment of video data is immediately followed by a segment of audio data), or have separate streams for video and audio (resulting in more processing and marginally larger files – DVEncoder 2).

MPEG

MPEG (Moving Pictures Experts Group – an ISO body) defines a compressed bit data stream, but the compression algorithms are up to individual manufacturers. MPEG-1 (roughly equivalent to VHS in quality) defines up to 1.5 megabits per second (consuming about 10 MB/min) whereas MPEG-2 (DVD standard) defines 3–10 megabits per second (consuming 20 to 70 MB/min). MPEG uses many of the same techniques as JPEG, but adds interframe compression to exploit similarities that occur between successive frames. It works by taking a relatively low resolution (352 by 288 pixel frames for MPEG-1; 720 by 576 for MPEG-2), 25 frames/second video in combination with high (compact disc) quality audio. The images are in colour, but are converted to YUV space (Y is the luma), and the two chrominance channels (U and V) are further reduced (to 176 by 144 pixel frames as resolution loss in these channels is less obvious – MPEG-1). Three types of coding are involved. Intraframes (I) code the still image. Predictive frames (P) predict motion from frame to frame (using discrete cosine transforms) to organize special redundancy (16×16 blocks in the 'Y' luminance channel). Lastly, the bidirectional (B) frames are predicted from the closest match in the last I or P frames. The audio compression (approximately 6:1, compared to approximately 26:1 for video) involves psychoacoustic modelling to remove the parts of sound least detectable by the human ear (e.g. masking effects will prevent a low energy sound being heard by the human ear if accompanied by a large component at a close by frequency).

Audio carried on MPEG movie format is now called MP3 – the popular music compression used in hand-held memory-based personal stereos. MP3 stands for MPEG-1, Audio Layer 3, and not MPEG-3 as the press sometime states. MPEG-3 was never developed as it was intended for professional use of MPEG-2, but instead MPEG-2 was extended. Nowadays there is also MPEG-4 (low bit rate video and object coding of video used in hand-held PDAs for video), MPEG-7 and MPEG-11 (both of which are tackling issues such as 'metadata').

Most movie files involve some form of compression to minimize their storage size. The compression algorithm is known as a codec and this must be installed by the program you wish to use to display your movie file. Codec is an abbreviation of 'coder/decoder', which describes a device or program capable of performing transformations on a data stream or signal. Codecs can both put the stream or signal into an encoded form (often for transmission, storage or encryption) and retrieve, or decode, that form for viewing or manipulation in a format more appropriate for these operations. Codecs are often used in videoconferencing and streaming media solutions (e.g. MPEG-4 Video). Many multimedia data streams contain audio, video and some form of metadata that permits synchronization of the audio and video which must be encapsulated together. The codec is not to be confused with the file format (or container) used to store the audio/video information encoded by the codec. File formats such as '.mpg', '.avi' and '.mov' are used to store information encoded by a codec. Programs designed specifically for displaying movie files, such as Windows Movie Player, will tend to have more intrinsic codecs than programs which can display movie files as one of their many functions such as Powerpoint. Most codecs are supplied with the hardware that utilizes them or can be downloaded from the World Wide Web.

Movie editing

As well as being able to take and store digital movies, it is important to be able to edit them. Taking a movie clip of exactly

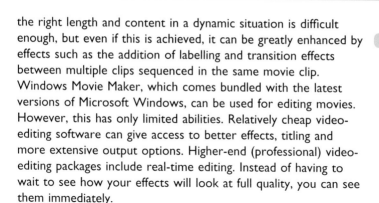

the right length and content in a dynamic situation is difficult enough, but even if this is achieved, it can be greatly enhanced by effects such as the addition of labelling and transition effects between multiple clips sequenced in the same movie clip. Windows Movie Maker, which comes bundled with the latest versions of Microsoft Windows, can be used for editing movies. However, this has only limited abilities. Relatively cheap video-editing software can give access to better effects, titling and more extensive output options. Higher-end (professional) video-editing packages include real-time editing. Instead of having to wait to see how your effects will look at full quality, you can see them immediately.

Most recent personal computers (PCs) are fast enough for video editing, but video editing is still one area where the quicker the PC the better. As well as a fast processor (greater than 2.0 GHz), you will need at least 512 MB of RAM (random access memory). RAM is the working memory of the computer and will greatly affect the speed of processing. Movie storage is memory hungry so you will need a lot of free hard disk space. It is worth considering a second internal or external hard disk, dedicated to video-editing files. Most movie software requires both the storage of your unedited movie and the workings of your editing before your final clip can be created. DV quality video requires 3.6 MB per second, or more than a gigabyte for a 5-minute video clip. A video card is no longer essential for video imaging. Video can be fed through the USB port either directly from the video camera or via an 'external' analogue-to-digital video-USB converter, but even USB2 has difficulties delivering full resolution DV quality at 25 Hz (standard PAL television quality). Many desktop PCs have FireWire ports as standard, but even if they do not, a PCI (Peripheral Component Interconnect) card that can be inserted into a slot on the side of your PC costs very little. A FireWire interface also allows you to control your video camera from the software rather than the controls on the camera itself.

Once you have loaded in your video, most editing packages allow you to edit using a time line or story board. A time line splits the movie into chunks (typically 10 seconds each or each separately recorded section on the video tape), which can be drawn down onto your editing palette and compressed from either or both ends (Fig. 3.4). On a story board you define the timings of the sections you wish to keep and sequence together (Fig. 3.5). Features that you may want to use in your video editing include the following:

- Sound stored with your video clip (if appropriate) can be cut or overwritten. The volume can be changed (such as fading in or out). Music tracks can be added and even fitted to automatically match the length of your video clip (actually a very complex musical process). As with your video, the audio can be encoded to save on disk space.
- Transitions can be added between sequences such as fades, wipes and even as advanced as the current image turning into a bird and flying into the following video sequence. Not only are these fun, but they give a movie sequence a more flowing professional feel. Some packages allow additional transitions to be purchased.
- Filters such as matte, chromaticity and luminance can be applied to the video.
- Picture-in-picture is the ability to edit a movie so that two or more video images are run simultaneously, usually one in a window overlaying the other. This is ideal for showing a close-up and overall view of a condition at the same time or an

Figure 3.4 Example of a movie-editing time line.

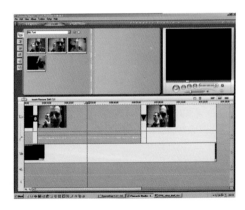

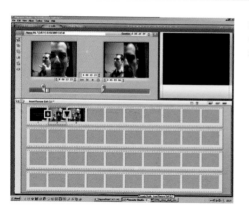

outside view of a piece of equipment being used and the internal view of what is seen by the user for a teaching movie. This feature requires the software to have good real-time rendering capabilities to prevent the output from skipping frames. For example, to help with complex portions, the software can use a buffer to render ahead of time during simpler sections.

- Editing and creation in different movie formats such as AVI, MPEG, MPEG-2 (based on the high-definition video format), QuickTime, RealMedia, Windows Medium Video (WMV), DV and uncompressed video and the ability to mix them within the same sequence.
- Output through USB or FireWire to put your edited clip onto a VHS tape or mini-DV tape or straight onto a television.
- Wizards to simplify frequent activities such as importing media or outputting video.
- Titling or labelling which can be overlaid on the video, or separate images or backgrounds with text inserted.
- DVD authoring so that a movie can be accessed at key points during its length or compact disc (CD) burning.

4
Anterior eye imaging

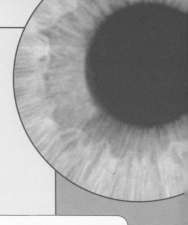

Slit-lamp biomicroscope system types

The slit-lamp biomicroscope is the most commonly used instrumentation in clinical practice to observe the anterior eye, allowing manipulation of the image enlargement and illumination (Fig. 4.1). As with retinal imaging, techniques such as using green (red-free) light for viewing blood vessels can enhance the captured image (Owen et al 2002). Image capture can allow automatic objective grading of anterior eye characteristics, such as hyperaemia and staining (Wolffsohn and Purslow 2003), corneal transparency (Polunin et al 1998, O'Donnell and

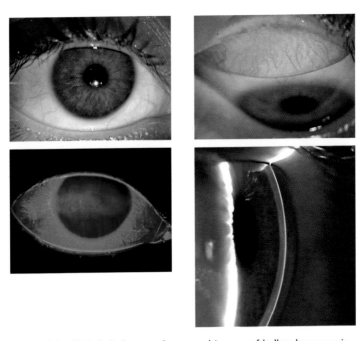

Figure 4.1 Digital slit-lamp and captured images of bulbar hyperaemia (top left), palpebral hyperaemia (top right), tear film with fluorescein instilled (bottom left) and a corneal section (bottom right). (From Wolffsohn and Peterson 2006, with permission.)

Wolffsohn 2004), lenticular opacification (Friedman et al 1999), and feature size and shape (Lin and Stern 1998). As with other digital imaging, the captured pictures can then be compressed and transmitted for teleophthalmic screening (Yogesan et al 1998; see Chapter 7).

Anterior segment imaging can be considered more skilled than retinal imaging as the operator needs to be skilled in slit-lamp biomicroscopy as well as photography.

The slit-lamp you choose to use for an imaging system is up to personal choice. There is a vast range of instruments available and these differ slightly in the features they offer. Along with the ability to alter the slit width (ideally with a calibrated control so the light beam width can be used to estimate the size of features noted) and height (ideally over a 14 mm range with incremental steps or variable calibrated scale down to 0.2 mm), a diffuser and yellow filter (see 'Fluorescein imaging' section on p. 57) are essential. For imaging, it is not important whether the slit-lamp biomicroscope has convergent or parallel eye-pieces, but as the binocularity of the instrument is necessary for assessment of depth, this characteristic should be considered, convergent eye-pieces being found by some to be more comfortable to use. The range of magnification should be approximately $5\times$ to $40\times$. Some prefer the continuous zoom with the ability to increase the magnification without interrupting the view of the object of interest. However, the optics cannot be as well optimized as the stepped dial approach with an individual set of optimized lenses for each magnification level. Calibration of images for measurement of distances and areas (see 'Image manipulation' section on p. 33) also requires the actual magnification that the image was taken with to be known, which is easier if only set magnification levels are on offer. As not all slit-lamp biomicroscopes have the option of retro-fitting of a beam splitter and cameras incorporated in the slit-lamp body are usually exclusive to a particular biomicroscope, future use of a slit-lamp biomicroscope should be considered on purchase, particularly any thoughts of upgrading to a photographic system, to save future expense due to incompatibility.

Camera attachments

There are three main options for anterior segment imaging with a slit-lamp biomicroscope.

1. Eye-piece attachment

This involves attaching a camera system to the existing eye-pieces of the slit-lamp (Fig. 4.2). The main advantage is the relatively low cost of such a system, although the expense of computer image database storage programs and image boards should not be forgotten. The slit-lamp eye-pieces have optics designed for the ~60 D cornea/lens assembly which have to be reversed to allow in-focus imaging by a camera (see 'Image manipulation' section on p. 33). Therefore the optical path is different from that of a purpose dedicated photographic slit-lamp. Light loss occurs at the eye-piece lens assembly, but an internal beam splitter is unnecessary. The field of view of the image is also generally reduced and the camera obscures at least

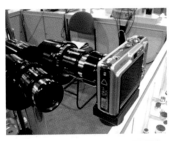
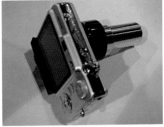
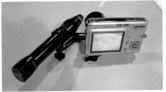
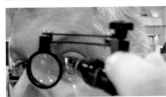

Figure 4.2 Eye-piece attachment camera examples. TTI digital camera to slit-lamp eye-piece adaptors are adaptable for most inside tube measurements (top). Hand-held slit-torch with camera attachment (bottom).

one eye-piece, so the advantages of a binocular system are lost in aligning and focusing an object of interest. Eye-pieces with a screw mounting (typically a C-mount) are available principally for Haag-Streit slit-lamps and can be attached to many different commercially available analogue and digital videos/cameras. The camera should be set for distance photography (usually depicted as mountains) to disable the automatic focus and flash. With the improvements in the imaging chips used in commercial video camcorders, these have also been used in conjunction with a screw mounting for connecting to slit-lamp eye-pieces and beam splitters. In general, few eye-piece attachment systems are available commercially, perhaps due to the relatively small profit margin that can be achieved with this option for anterior eye imaging.

2. Attached to a beam splitter

This involves a beam splitter being inserted into the optical path of the slit-lamp with a camera attached (Fig. 4.3). Most photo slit-lamps on the market are of this form and a beam-splitter module can be added to many medium to high quality slit-lamps. The beam splitter can be dropped into place when imaging functionality is required, but removed when only eye-piece examination is necessary to maximize the image light intensity available to the clinician. The use of a beam splitter still allows binocular viewing through the eye-pieces and hence the camera only receives ~50% (depending on the reflectance of the beam splitter) of the available light. To date, no companies market a mirror system module, which would increase the light sensitivity of the photo slit-lamp by a factor of approximately two, still allowing focusing using the video monitor (but not through the eye-pieces).

3. Integrated into the slit-lamp

These are similar in principle to those described for option 2, but the beam splitter and camera are built into a single unit which can generally only be attached to one slit-lamp. This creates a neater imaging solution and limits the number of cables required from the camera to the computer; hence they are a

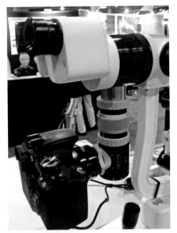
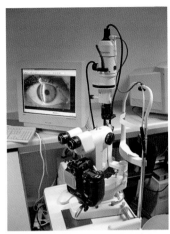
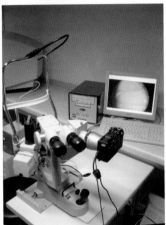
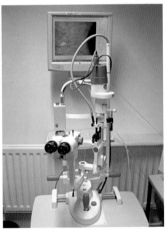

Figure 4.3 Beam splitter attachment and digital camera examples (TTI beam splitter; Zeiss Canon G3; Topcon Nikon D1X and Carleton/ARC Jai SV3500).

popular option for using on combi-units and where the consulting room already has a computer controlling the test chart, fundus camera or patient management system (Fig. 4.4). However, the integrated slit-lamp image capture system does restrict the owner to the manufacturer's camera products (which

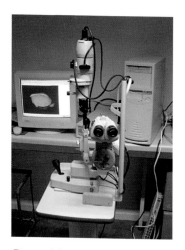 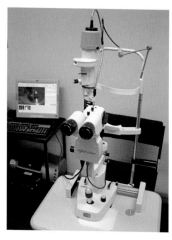

Figure 4.4 Integrated slit-lamp imaging system examples (Topcon DC1 and CSO Digital Vision).

may not keep up with the advances or cost-competitiveness of commercial digital cameras) and could cause maintenance problems if the camera becomes damaged or faulty and the practice is reliant on the basic slit-lamp biomicroscope. In addition to an integrated slit-lamp capture system, the use of compact computers (sometimes referred to as 'cubes') helps to reduce the system footprint.

Cameras

There are many camera options available, as highlighted on page 11. The continuously refreshed real-time image viewed on a monitor shows exactly what can be captured in terms of image focus, contrast, illuminance and field of view. Discrepancies in these image characteristics are common between the image viewed through the slit-lamp eye-piece(s) and that captured by the attached camera, especially with photographic systems reliant on a flash unit and the observer's involuntary accommodation through the eye-pieces (Hammack 1995). As mentioned previously, this was the main problem with previous photographic methods, even to an extent with Polaroid cameras if an image was difficult to set up, or you had limited time with a patient. Therefore, a real-time monitor image is critical to good imaging.

Analogue PAL or NTSC composite video cameras (see p. 17), typically with resolutions around 0.5 megapixels, are cheap and can provide up to 25 or 30 interlaced images a second (25 Hz or 30 Hz, respectively). Digital cameras can capture images at much higher resolutions than analogue cameras, but they are generally more expensive, have a slower refresh rate and require more complex (and therefore more expensive) image capture cards. Although commercially available digital cameras often have a small built-in real-time monitor, this is generally inadequate to allow non-eye-piece focusing of the image. However, an analogue output is usually available and can be fed into a larger monitor to allow subjective manipulation of the slit-lamp to produce the optimum captured image. Single lens reflex (SLR) cameras have the advantage of allowing the user to see exactly what the lens is capturing, but divert light away from the sensor towards the eye-piece when the camera viewfinder is being used, preventing a simultaneous live video feed (Fig. 4.5). Features such as autofocusing must be disabled from commercial cameras, usually by selecting infinity ('mountain') viewing.

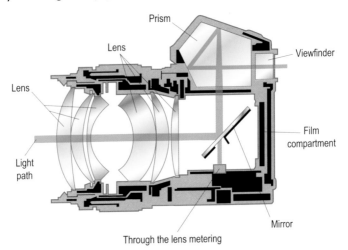

Figure 4.5 Imaging mechanism of a single lens reflex camera.

Resolution

Two of the major considerations with digital imaging are the resolution needed to image the object of interest and the compression that can be utilized to minimize the space needed to store the image (Charman 1998). If photographs are to be used to detect pathology, monitor progression and protect against litigation, it is essential that the resolution is sufficient to allow all clinical features of interest to be detected and that this is not compromised by the image storage. Resolution is the ability to distinguish the difference between two sequential points. In digital imagery, this depends on the number of pixels that the image is composed of (Jensen and Scherfig 1999). Peterson and Wolffsohn (2005) examined the theoretical and clinical minimum image pixel resolution and maximum compression appropriate for anterior eye image storage.

The smallest objects of clinical relevance observed by slit-lamp microscopy on the anterior eye were considered to be microcysts and punctate staining. Microcysts have been reported as being 15–50 µm in diameter (Zantos 1983, Keay et al 2001, Tabery 2003). Therefore it seems appropriate that digital imaging should detect an object of ~30 µm in diameter. As the light from an object could fall across the diameter of two pixels, a pixel size equivalent to 15 µm is necessary for reliable image capture. As the magnification (and hence the field of view) of a slit-lamp image can be varied, a typical slit-lamp imaging system was used to calculate the necessary horizontal resolution of a digital camera to be able to reliably detect an object of 30 µm (ARC, Carleton, Chesham, UK; Table 4.1). For example, theoretical calculation suggested that the minimum resolution should be $\geq$579 horizontal pixels at 25× magnification.

Clinical images of the bulbar conjunctiva, palpebral conjunctiva and corneal staining were taken at the maximum resolution of four cameras attached to the same Takagi slit-lamp (Nagano-Ken, Japan) in turn. The images were stored in TIFF format and further copies created with reduced resolution (Fig. 4.6). The images were then ranked for clarity on a 15-inch monitor (resolution 1280 × 1024) by 20 practitioners and analysed by objective image

Table 4.1 Resolution necessary to detect an object of interest of size 30 μm with varying typical slit-lamp magnifications

Slit lamp magnification	Horizontal field of view (μm)	Resolution necessary to detect 30 μm object
40×	5 590	≥373 pixels
25×	8 950	≥597 pixels
16×	13 980	≥932 pixels
10×	22 365	≥1491 pixels
6.3×	35 500	≥2367 pixels

analysis grading. Subjective grading identified that an image could be reduced to 767 × 569 pixel resolution (an 88% reduction in file size compared to a 2048 × 1360 pixel image) with no perceivable loss in image quality and this was independent of the camera used to take the images. As the screen resolution of the monitor that was used to view the images was 1280 × 1024, it is not surprising that high resolution images did not offer any improvement in apparent image quality. Instead the necessary integration of pixels to display the higher resolution image on the screen led to a perceived reduction in image quality. Objective grading (see 'Objective image analysis' section on p. 67) was less susceptible to resolution degradation, such that images could be reduced up to 640 × 425 pixel resolution with no significant change in edge detection grading, and even a reduction to 160 × 107 pixels had no effect on colour extraction.

Table 4.2 displays the average file sizes of the three images and four cameras for the different levels of resolution utilized and the percentage difference from maximum image quality. A reduction in resolution to 767 × 569 pixels, which was shown to cause no appreciable subjective image degradation on a computer screen, caused an 88% reduction in file size.

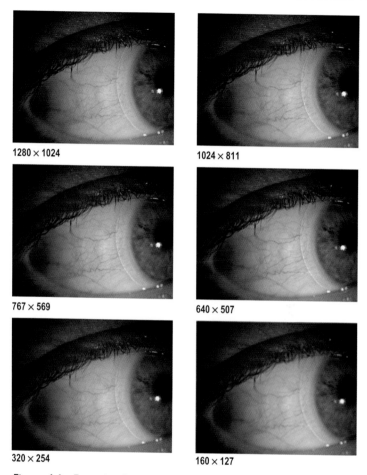

1280 × 1024

1024 × 811

767 × 569

640 × 507

320 × 254

160 × 127

Figure 4.6 Example of an image saved at a range of resolutions.

Fluorescein imaging

Fluorescein is a vital dye (i.e. it can be used in vivo in human eyes); on absorbing blue light (optimally around 485 nm), its molecules are excited to a higher state and fluoresce light of a

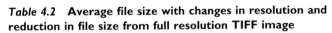

Table 4.2 Average file size with changes in resolution and reduction in file size from full resolution TIFF image

TIFF pixel resolution	File size (MB)	Reduction (%)
2048 × 1360	8656.7	0
1600 × 1063	4393.3	49.3
1280 × 811	2198.3	74.6
1024 × 680	1670.0	80.7
767 × 569	1041.3	88.0
640 × 425	621.3	92.8
320 × 213	231.1	97.3
160 × 107	75.5	99.1

higher wavelength (around 510–520 nm appearing green; Fig. 4.7). The fluorescent dye can enter the eye via either systemic administration (intravenous injection or ingestion) or topical administration to the cornea. The dye mixes with the surrounding fluid (blood or tears), highlighting its dynamics (such as tear break-up time) and volume. The concentration of fluorescein remaining in a sample of the tear film 15 minutes after instillation (measured by fluorophotometry), or in the lateral tear meniscus 2 minutes after instillation (assessed against a grading scale), is correlated to ocular irritation symptoms and eyelid and corneal disease (Macri et al 2000). Fluorescein can be used to assess the fit of rigid gas-permeable contact lenses (Costa and Franco 1998). Fluorescein diffuses into intercellular spaces, such as defects in the tight junctions (zonulae occludens) of the basal epithelial cells or cell drop-out, resulting in staining. Fluorescein cannot penetrate intact cell membranes, but once fluorescein gains entry it diffuses freely to the interior of surrounding cells by passing through junctional surfaces (Romanchuk 1982).

To clearly view the fluorescent light, it is important that this is not obscured by reflected blue light from the ocular surface used

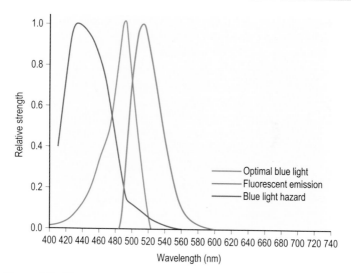

Figure 4.7 The optimal blue light spectrum for exciting fluorescein and the resulting fluorescein emission, together with the blue light hazard. (Adapted McLaren and Brubaker (1983), with permission.)

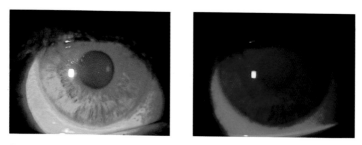

Figure 4.8 An eye illuminated by blue light with (right) and without (left) a yellow fluorescein enhancement filter placed in the observation system.

to stimulate the fluorescein molecules. This is best achieved by the placement of a yellow barrier filter, with minimal transmission below 500 nm and maximum above this level, in the observation system (Fig. 4.8). Although often called a Wratten filter, Wratten is just the name of a set of filters made by Kodak with a wide range of spectral profiles (only a few of which are yellow in colour – Wratten 12 being the most appropriate) so this is an inappropriate name to use for fluorescein barrier filters.

As well as having an excitatory light source of sufficient power at the wavelengths absorbed by the fluorophore and minimal power at wavelengths emitted by fluorescence of the fluorophore, exposing the eye to light in the range of damaging blue light should be minimized (Fig. 4.7). Blue light can damage the eye if of high enough intensities and long enough duration (Margrain et al 2004). Slit-lamps used clinically for macular imaging can produce enough light to exceed the maximum permissible exposure in <15 seconds (Calkins et al 1980). McLaren and Brubaker (1983) examined a range of different light sources in combination with barrier filters for their fluorescein excitation and blue light hazard, identifying an argon laser to be the most suitable light source, although tungsten filaments used traditionally in slit-lamp biomicroscopes were ranked second with a safe exposure time for a 3.0×0.2 mm slit on the retina of ~70 minutes.

Fortunately the optimal blue light for anterior eye fluorescein viewing does not alter with the pH of tears. The emission spectra of fluorescein changes in magnitude, but not spectral profile, with solution pH in the range of 6 to 9 (Wang and Gaigalas 2002). The intensity of fluorescence increases with increasing pH, reaches a plateau at approximately pH 8 and then decreases with further increases in pH (Romanchuk 1982). A higher tear film pH will result in a higher fluorescent output, although the peak absorption wavelength remains relatively unaffected. The pH in the conjunctival sac is typically 6.93 ± 0.27 (range 5.9–7.6), independent of age and gender (Norn 1988). The conjunctival fluid is significantly more acid in contact lens wearers (by ~0.2 on average), but becomes normalized after lens removal. The conjunctival fluid pH is relatively unaffected by most anterior conditions, but is significantly more alkaline in patients with fungal keratitis (7.40 ± 0.23), 1 day post corneal graft (7.21 ± 0.22) and dry eyes (7.13 ± 0.31; Norn 1988).

Peterson et al (2006) examined the spectral radiance output of slit-lamp blue illumination and the spectral transmission of yellow barrier enhancement filters. They showed that few currently available slit-lamps had a blue light source that was optimal for fluorescein viewing and imaging (Fig. 4.9) and that yellow filters typically had a cut-off wavelength that was too high, removing about two-thirds of the fluorescein fluoresced light (Fig. 4.10).

The intensity of fluorescence of fluorescein in aqueous solution increases with increasing concentration up to a maximum (approximately 0.001–0.04%) and then falls off at higher concentrations (termed quenching; Romanchuk 1982). At higher concentrations, the maximum emission spectrum is shifted towards longer wavelengths (more yellow than green). The intensity of fluorescence observed is also related to the depth of fluorescein solution and the angle of the incident light (Romanchuk 1982). All fluorescein instillation techniques cause some initial quenching during the tear mixing process. A moistened Fluoret and the 1% Minims reach a useful level of fluorescence in on average ~20 s and this lasts for ~160 s,

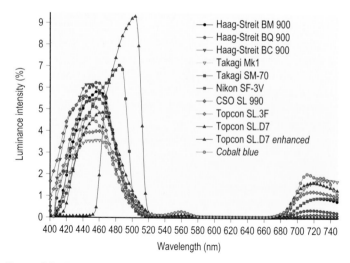

Figure 4.9 Blue light emission of slit-lamp biomicroscopes currently available. Note the difference between the more ideal spectra and that of cobalt blue. (Redrawn from Peterson et al 2006, with permission.)

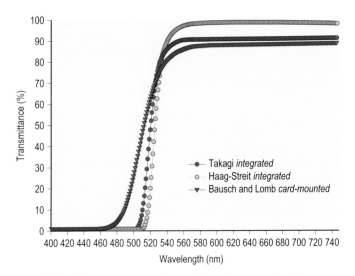

Figure 4.10 Light transmission from slit-lamp integrated and cardboard-mounted yellow fluorescein enhancement filters. (Redrawn from Peterson et al 2006, with permission.)

although a 1% Minims gives a greater fluorescent intensity (Fig. 4.11). In comparison, saturated Fluorets and 2% Minims take ~2.5 times as long to reach useful fluorescence, for little additional duration. Therefore instillation of fluorescein using a moistened Fluoret or 1% Minims is most appropriate clinically (Peterson et al 2006).

Illumination techniques

One of the main advantages of slit-lamp viewing of the anterior eye is the flexibility of the illumination system to optimize viewing of the feature of interest. The slit height, width, intensity orientation and position relative to the camera centre (decoupling) can be manipulated. Often several types of illumination are evident at the same time, as the field of view of the observation system is larger than the area illuminated by the

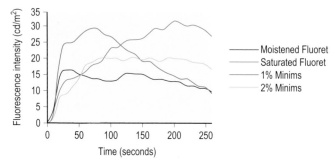

Figure 4.11 Fluorescence resulting from instillation of fluorescein by drop or Fluoret with time. (Redrawn from Peterson et al 2006, with permission.)

slit. Moving the illumination and/or observation across the anterior eye surface applies a range of illumination techniques to each area, highlighting disturbances to the expected appearance. There are seven main illumination techniques.

1. Diffuse

The illumination is spread evenly over the anterior eye surface to allow general low magnification examination of the external eye and adnexa (Fig. 4.12).

2. Direct illumination

A slit of light is viewed directly illuminating the area of interest. The slit is narrowed to produce an optic section which is orientated perpendicular to the cornea, with the observation system positioned obliquely to view the depth of corneal incursions and the anterior chamber, and to observe the main corneal layers (Fig. 4.13). Parallelepiped illumination is a wider optic section, reducing the ability to differentiate depth, but assisting in observing a wider field. For viewing cells (seen as flare due to the Tyndall effect) caused by inflammation of the anterior chamber, a slit beam of minimal height is shone through the pupil at an angle to the observation system in a dark room (conic beam).

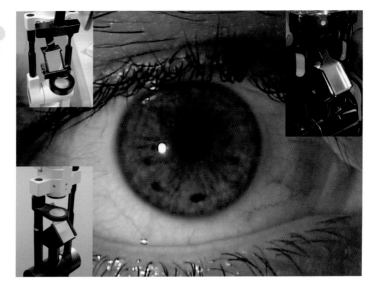

Figure 4.12 Diffuse illumination and a range of diffusing systems.

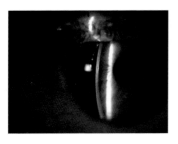
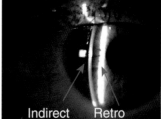

Indirect   Retro

Figure 4.13 Direct illumination as an optic section (top left), parallelepiped (top right) and conic beam (bottom right) with areas of indirect and retro-illumination indicated.

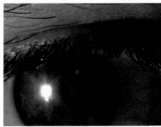

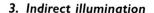
3. Indirect illumination
This can highlight features obscured by direct illumination and is observation to the side of a direct beam (Fig. 4.13). To centre the indirect illumination, the slit-lamp illumination system needs to be decoupled.

4. Retro-illumination
This is back illumination created by reflecting the light off a surface. Usually the cornea is observed with light reflected off the iris or retina (Fig. 4.13). Again, the illumination needs to be uncoupled from the observation system to centre the area of retro-illumination.

5. Specular reflection
This occurs when the angles of illumination and observation are equal and opposite about the axis normal to a surface. This creates a Purkinje image wherever there is a change in refractive index. For the cornea:

- Purkinje I – the front surface of the tear film. The tears can be seen moving just to the side of the bright reflection after a blink.
- Purkinje II – the endothelium. The endothelial mosaic of hexagonal cells can be seen under high (~40×) magnification in the dimmer reflection.
- Purkinje III – front surface of the lens. A dimpled appearance can be seen with quite a narrow angle between the observation and illumination system (Fig. 4.14).

6. Sclerotic scatter
The illumination slit is decoupled and rotated onto the limbus. Total internal reflection diverts the light through the cornea, creating a halo around the rest of the limbus where the light exits the cornea (Fig. 4.15). If there is an opacity or irregularity in the cornea (such as oedema induced by rigid contact lenses), the internal light path will be disrupted and the discrepancy highlighted.

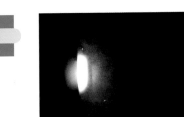
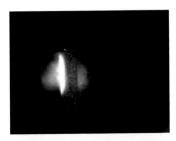
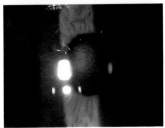

Figure 4.14 Specular reflection illumination of the tear film (top left), endothelial corneal cells (top right) and crystalline lens surface (bottom right).

Figure 4.15 Sclerotic scatter illumination of the cornea.

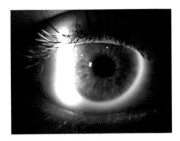

7. Tangential illumination

The illumination system is set parallel to the iris and observed along the visual axis. It can be useful in inspecting the iris for raised areas such as naevi. It is difficult to achieve using the slit-lamp observation system in most cases, as in order to traverse the iris surface with the illumination system the slit-lamp has to be too far forward to allow in-focus viewing of the result.

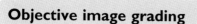

Objective image grading

The current best practice for the assessment and recording of anterior eye features is in the form of subjective grading scales which were introduced to reduce inconsistencies between examiners and to encourage uniform grading of the anterior eye (Efron 1998, Fieguth and Simpson 2002, Efron et al 2001). The level on the scale (commonly four to five predetermined images) that best matches the characteristic of the eye under observation is recorded, ideally to one decimal place to improve discrimination (Bailey et al 1991). However, these scales remain (by their nature) subjective and lead to inherently variable assessments with a wide range of the scale utilized by different practitioners to describe the same image (Fieguth and Simpson 2002, Wolffsohn 2004). Practitioners also demonstrate a reluctance to interpolate between the grading images displayed, even if training has been undertaken (Efron et al 2003). This is compounded by the design of the scales themselves which are not linear in nature, instead having increased sensitivity at the lower end, although this is not always consistent (Wolffsohn 2004).

To improve this situation various studies have investigated computer-based *objective* grading of ocular surfaces. With respect to vascular changes, several parameters have been the focus of objective analysis software (Papas 2000, Wolffsohn and Purslow 2003). Edge detection and colour extraction have been shown to be the most repeatable and discriminatory of those techniques (Wolffsohn and Purslow 2003), and have been found to be up to 50× more sensitive (up to 0.02 of an Efron unit) and 16× more reliable than subjective grading (Fig. 4.16). Objective image analysis of the anterior eye therefore offers a new gold-standard in anterior ocular examination and could be developed further as a tool for use in research, to allow more highly powered analysis without bias, and in clinical practice to enhance the monitoring of anterior eye disease.

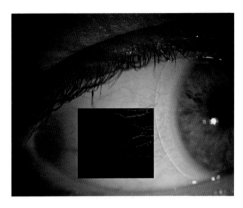

Figure 4.16 Edge detection of the bulbar conjunctiva by image analysis. The selected area red coloration compared to the combined red, green and blue colour intensity is also analysed as part of the objective grading. The same technique can be applied to other anterior eye features such as palpebral hyperaemia, palpebral roughness and the area of staining.

Scheimpflug technique

The Scheimpflug principle images the anterior eye with a camera at an angle to a slit-beam creating an optic section of the cornea and lens (Fig. 4.17). It has been used for the assessment of cataract (Hockwin et al 1984, Wegener and Laser 2001), intraocular lens shape changes with accommodation (Dubbelman et al 2003), corneal haze (Smith et al 1990, Soya et al 2002, van de Pol et al 2001), corneal curvature and corneal thickness (Morgan et al 2002). More recent instrumentation has been designed to rotate around the visual axis capturing multiple images to create a three-dimensional image of the anterior chamber. Scheimpflug measures of central corneal thickness and anterior chamber depth have been shown to have good repeatability compared to Orbscan topography, ultrasonography and MRI (Koretz et al 2004, Lackner et al 2005, Hashemi et al 2005).

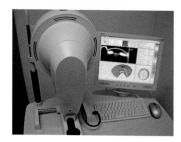
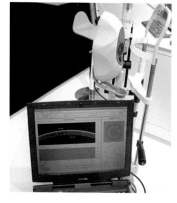

Figure 4.17 Scheimpflug devices showing captured images of the anterior eye. (From Wolffsohn and Peterson 2006, with permission.)

Corneal topography

Topography is particularly important in clinical practice for fitting contact lenses to irregular corneas, detecting and monitoring corneal pathological conditions such as keratoconus and pellucid marginal degeneration and assessing the effects of laser refractive surgery and penetrating keratoplasty. It can inform laser retreatments, the removal of sutures and postoperative fitting of contact lenses. Topography is the assessment of shape, whereas tomography relates to sectioning through an object.

Using the cornea as a convex mirror, the size of the reflection of a known dimension light source at a set distance can be measured and used to calculate the topography of the front surface of the cornea (Fig. 4.18). Usually multiple light concentric rings are reflected off the cornea (reflection system) and the image captured by a central camera (Placido disc). The image is transferred to a computer image capture board, with the position of the reflected rings analysed and displayed as colour-coded isobars of corneal radius or power. Alternatively, a slit beam of light can be passed across the cornea (projection system) and imaged multiple times at an offset angle (in a similar

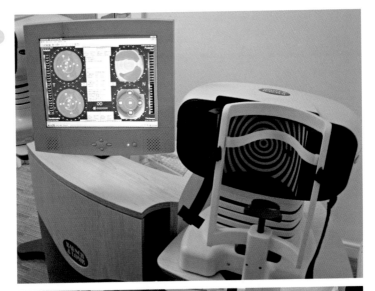

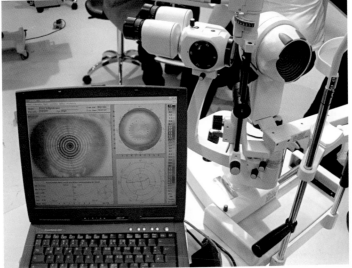

Figure 4.18 Raster (top) and Placido (bottom) topographers showing contour maps of the cornea. (From Wolffsohn and Peterson 2006, with permission.)

manner to Scheimpflug imaging) to quantify the curvature of both the front and back surface of the cornea, together with the corneal thickness (know as raster topography or posterior apical radius imaging; Liu et al 1999). The accuracy and reproducibility is similar to Placido-based systems (approximately 4 μm in the central cornea and 7 μm in the periphery under optimal conditions), but the technique does not require an intact epithelial surface (Mejia-Barbosa and Malacara-Hernandez 2001). However, due to the longer capture time for the multiple images, it is more dependent than Placido-based corneal topography on factors such as the patient's fixation and ability to keep the eye open.

Curvature/power maps

In interpreting the results clinically, it is important to differentiate between absolute and normalized maps. Absolute maps have a preset colour scale with the same radius or power steps, maximum and minimum assigned to the same colours for the particular instrument. These maps allow direct comparison of two different maps, but the large increments between steps (typically 0.5 D) mask small localized changes in curvature, such as early keratoconus. Normalized maps, on the other hand, cover the scale range of the particular cornea being assessed. Therefore they tend to have smaller step increments and show more detail, but the colour scale is not comparable to other topography maps.

1. **Axial curvature** (also known as sagittal curvature) displays the curvature at each point on the corneal surface in axial direction relative to the (presumed) centre. The axial value at a point on the cornea is equal to the average meridional curvature from that point along the radius to the map centre, thereby approximating the average refractive power.
2. **Tangential curvature** (also know as instantaneous or meridional curvature) displays the curvature at each point on the corneal surface in meridional direction relative to the other points on the particular ring.

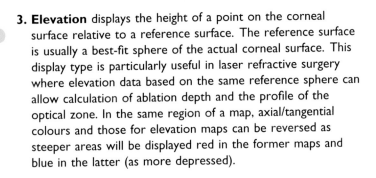

3. **Elevation** displays the height of a point on the corneal surface relative to a reference surface. The reference surface is usually a best-fit sphere of the actual corneal surface. This display type is particularly useful in laser refractive surgery where elevation data based on the same reference sphere can allow calculation of ablation depth and the profile of the optical zone. In the same region of a map, axial/tangential colours and those for elevation maps can be reversed as steeper areas will be displayed red in the former maps and blue in the latter (as more depressed).

Topographic indexes

1. **Simulated K values** simulate traditional keratometer readings by expressing the curvature in two orthogonal axes (90° apart) in the central ~3 mm area of the cornea.
2. **Index of asphericity** indicates how much the corneal curvature changes from the centre to the periphery of the cornea. A normal cornea is prolate (i.e. becomes flatter toward the periphery). Various parameters have been used to describe corneal asphericity, the most common of which are related to each other such that $Q = p - 1 = -e^2$ (Gatinel et al 2002).

Errors in the topographical mapping of the cornea can occur from a disrupted epithelial surface or tear film, inaccurate focusing or alignment of the instrument or poor patient fixation, and the dependence of each point on the accuracy of the more central points, leading to increased inaccuracy toward the periphery. Complex irregular corneal surfaces, such as those from keratoconus, can lead to large measurement errors (McMahon et al 2005).

Confocal microscopy

Conventional microscopes collect all the light reflected back from an object, with blurred light from out of the focal plane resulting in optical noise, limiting the resolution of the technique. Therefore, objects of interest need to be thinly sliced to improve resolution, thus not applicable to in-vivo imaging. In confocal microscopy, the pinhole source of light (such as a laser beam) and its conjugate pinhole detector limit the out-of-focus signal that is collected (Fig. 4.19). However, the field of view is small and scanning is used to create a larger field image. The scanning is usually achieved by rotating discs with multiple optically conjugate source-detector pinholes. Confocal microscopy has a resolution of approximately 1 μm and a maximal imaging depth of about 2.7 mm, which allows it to image cells of the corneal epithelium, epithelial nerve plexus, different parts of the stroma, and endothelium. In-vivo corneal confocal microscopy can be used to make direct observations on living tissue, avoiding the shrinkage and distortion associated with conventional processing and sectioning for light microscopy (Freegard 1997). Confocal microscopy has improved understanding of the function of each of the corneal layers and their spatial location (Bohnke and Masters 1999) and has been extensively used to evaluate the progression and healing of inflammation or infection over time (Cavanagh et al 2000, Tervo and Moilanen 2003, Popper et al 2004). Confocal microscopy through focusing (CMTF) has been used in photorefractive surgery to assess corneal thickness, photoablation depth assessment and corneal light scatter (Moller-Pedersen et al 1997). However, confocal microscopy is limited to the assessment of a small area of the central cornea, which reduces its efficacy.

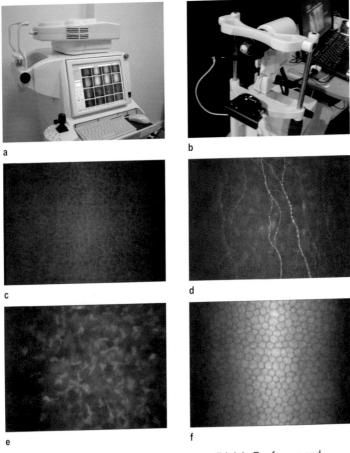

Figure 4.19 **(a, b)** Confocal microscopes (Nidek Confoscan and Haag-Streit HRT attachment) showing captured images of the epithelium **(c)**, Bowman's lamina **(d)**, stroma **(e)** and endothelium **(f)**. (From Wolffsohn and Peterson 2006, with permission.)

Optical coherence tomography

Optical coherence tomography (OCT) is a non-invasive optical method allowing cross-sectional imaging at a resolution of

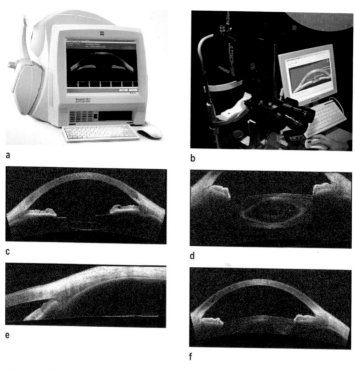

a

b

c

d

e

f

Figure 4.20 (a, b) Optical coherence tomographers (Zeiss Visante and Heidelberg systems) showing the anterior chamber (c), the crystalline lens (d), an intraocular lens and anterior capsulorhexis (e), and the ciliary body (f).

6–25 μm (Fig. 4.20). Ultrahigh resolution OCT with a spatial resolution of 1.3 μm can now be achieved (Reiser et al 2005). This allows imaging of the corneal layers and their thickness to be measured. It works by detecting the reflection of light from a structure in a similar way to how ultrasound uses sound, but as the speed of light is so much faster than sound (approximately 872 000 times) the reflection is assessed by interference. Laser light has a coherence length of many metres and as this dictates the axial resolution, a coherence length of micrometres is achieved by using a broadband light source such as super luminescent diode or short pulse (femtosecond) laser. The light source is split into a reference and measurement beam. Light from the measurement beam is reflected from the ocular structures and interacts with the reference light reflected from the reference mirror causing interference. Coherent (positive) interference, from where there is a reflection of light within the coherence length, is measured by an interferometer to allow an image of the reflected light from the ocular structures to be built up (Hirano et al 2001). Any light that is outside the short coherence length will not contribute to the coherence pattern.

In time domain OCT, a reflectivity profile (A-scan) is built by the reference mirror physically scanning over the coherence length. The mechanical action of the reference arm limits the potential resolution and clarity of image of time domain OCT. Spectral OCT overcomes the requirement to oscillate the reference mirror, creating broadband interference by spectrally separating the detectors, either by using a dispersive detector, such as a grating or a linear detector array, or by encoding the optical frequency in time with a spectrally scanning or 'swept' source (Choma et al 2003, Chen et al 2005). The A-scan is then calculated from the Fourier-transform of the acquired spectra. The imaging speed is improved and there are potential improvements in the signal-to-noise ratio proportional to the number of detector (silicon imaging chip) detection elements (pixels). The fall off in signal-to-noise ratio with penetration depth with dispersive detector OCT is overcome by using a swept source, although it has been suggested there are non-linearities with wavelength, especially at high scanning frequencies (Yasuno et al 2005). A cross-sectional tomograph (B-scan) may be achieved by laterally combining a series of axial depth scans (A-scan). As with any image recreation technique where a wave such as light or sound passes through curved media of differing refractive indices, the image needs to be compensated for these distortions to allow spatially accurate presentation and measurement.

In anterior eye imaging, OCT has been used to measure tear film thickness (Hirano et al 2001, King-Smith et al 2000, Wang et al 2003), and to examine the cornea and limbus (Feng and Simpson 2005), intraocular lens parameters, anterior chamber depth and the irido-corneal angle, even behind an opaque cornea

(Baikoff et al 2005). OCT can penetrate the human sclera in vivo, allowing high resolution, cross-sectional imaging of the anterior chamber angle and the ciliary body (Hoerauf et al 2002). However, the typical 1310 nm wavelength light is blocked by pigment, preventing exploration behind the iris (Baikoff et al 2005).

Ultrasonography

Ultrasonography uses high frequency mechanical pulses, usually generated by piezoelectric components, rather than light to assess the biometry of the anterior eye; the time for the reflected sound to return can be used to build up a picture of the front of the eye (Fig. 4.21). A-scan ultrasonography along the optical axis allows assessment of corneal thickness, anterior chamber depth, lens thickness and axial length. B-scan ultrasonography scans across the eye, allowing an image of the ocular structures to be built up. It has a precision of approximately 0.1 mm, but only moderately high intra-observer and low inter-observer reproducibility (Urbak 1998, 1999, Urbak et al 1998). It is an invasive technique and has reduced in popularity due to the commercialization of a partial-coherent interferometry device for measuring axial length and calculating intraocular lens power, which has a spatial resolution of approximately 0.01 mm and excellent reproducibility (Santodomingo-Rubido et al 2002). However, the latter cannot penetrate dense cataract as well as ultrasonography (Freeman and Pesudovs 2005). The resolution and depth of penetration of ultrasonography are affected by transducer frequency. Traditional ultrasonography of the whole eye uses a 10–20 MHz transducer, with approximately 100 µm resolution achieving 25 mm penetration. High frequency ultrasound biomicroscopy (UBM) with a transducer of approximately 50 MHz increases the tissue resolution to 30–50 µm, but reduces tissue penetration depth to 4–5 mm, which is still sufficient to image the anterior segment (Pavline et al 1990, 1992). As the technique uses high frequency pulses rather than light waves, it can penetrate opaque corneas to examine the ciliary body and surrounding structures.

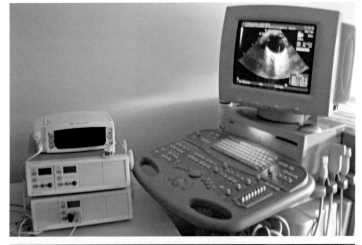

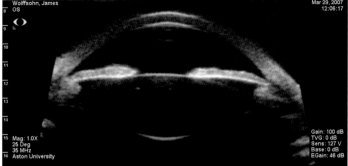

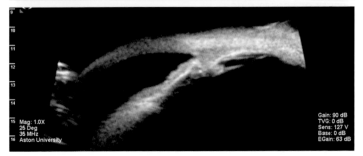

Figure 4.21 Ultrasound unit showing anterior eye sections.

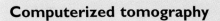
Computerized tomography

Computerized tomography (CT or CAT) emits several simultaneous X-rays from different angles. X-rays have high energy and short wavelength and are able to pass through tissue. The beams, which will be weaker if they have passed through dense tissue, are detected after they have passed through the body creating a cross-sectional image. CT scans are far more detailed than ordinary X-rays. A liquid X-ray dye can be injected into the veins during the test to enhance organs, blood vessels or tumours. Far more X-rays are involved in a CT scan than in ordinary X-rays, increasing the potential side effects, and some patients experience side effects due to allergic reactions to the liquid dye injected into the veins. For the eye, CT scans are usually used to assess ocular trauma, especially if a metal foreign body is suspected in which case MRI is contraindicated (Kolk et al 2005). However, CT may not differentiate whether the foreign body has penetrated the cornea and visibility will depend on the foreign body material (Deramo et al 1998).

Magnetic resonance imaging

Magnetic resonance imaging (MRI) uses electromagnetic waves combined with the reception of weak radio signals to record the density or concentration of hydrogen (or other) nuclei in the body (Charman 1998). MRI avoids health risks associated with ionizing radiation found in routine X-rays and CT scans, but can penetrate the whole human body. Furthermore, the resolution is greater than that of traditional CT scanning. The images of an MRI are reconstructed into cross-sections of anatomy (Fig. 4.22). In ophthalmology, MRI has been used to examine the whole eye and orbit with respect to space-occupying lesions, soft tissue damage and extraocular muscle examination (Kolk et al 2005, Ben Simon et al 2005, Sa et al 2005). It has also been used to study eye shape with refractive error and the crystalline lens changes with eye focus (Atchison et al 2004, Jones et al 2005).

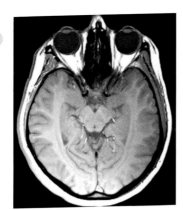

Figure 4.22 **(a)** Magnetic resonance imager head section across the ocular globe. **(b)** High resolution T1 scan of the eyes highlighting the ocular tissue. **(c)** High resolution T2 scan of the eyes highlighting the ocular fluids. (From Wolffsohn and Peterson 2006, with permission.)

a

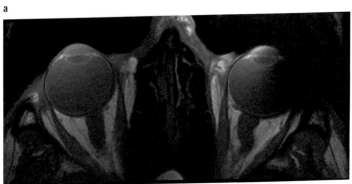

b

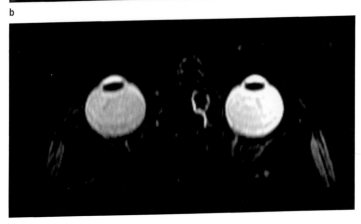

c

5
Posterior eye imaging

Fundus cameras

Fundus cameras have been available for many years. Traditional film-based systems had additional 'consumable' costs, for example the film and its processing (see p. 8). There was also the significant delay between capturing an image and being able to view it. This resulted in variable image quality and reduced efficiency in clinical care. Most retinal cameras now use digital imaging, allowing for images to be taken and instantaneously viewed. This offers the benefits of immediate determination of the most appropriate luminance to be used (see p. 9) and enables the viewer to maximize image positioning and clarity before capture. It is interesting to note that although the Glasgow workshop of the National Screening Committee recommended the use of digital photography as better for diabetic screening than film, Polaroid and dilated ophthalmoscopy (Fransen et al 2002, Ryder et al 1998, Bursell et al 2001, Lin et al 2002), not all studies have shown similar results (Lim et al 2000, AlSabti et al 2003).

Image capture

Fundus cameras image the fundus through the pupil. Most cameras show an initial, dynamic, black and white image of the pupil to allow alignment. Some allow the initial working distance to be more accurately determined using a split pupil presentation. A high positive powered lens is then dropped into place (some systems with quite an audible clunk) to neutralize the optical power of the crystalline lens and cornea, allowing an inverted aerial view of the fundus to be seen. This, again, is usually a black and white image as the lack of light filters to allow colour image processing (see 'Capture technology' section in Chapter 2) enables an image with lower light levels (more light-sensitive imager). A new retinal camera (Zeiss Visucam C; Fig. 5.1) simultaneously displays the live fundus image and also a miniaturized image of the external eye, which is used to aid alignment during infrared illumination. The Visucam C can also

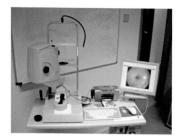 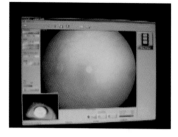

Figure 5.1 Zeiss Visucam C with its movie clip and dual image facility.

display and record a live dynamic (~12 Hz) colour movie clip of the anterior eye or fundus, enabling dynamic assessment of retinal and anterior eye conditions. This function can encourage patient interaction. Retinal cameras usually have markers overlaid on the fundus image to achieve accurate alignment and focusing of the image. 'Non-mydriatic' cameras are designed to allow a complete (usually 45°) image, through an undilated pupil. This works well in practice, although patients with very small pupils require careful alignment to prevent black shadows at the edges of the image.

Optics

As with anterior eye cameras, the optics of the camera are essential to gaining a high quality image. However, a fundus image is also reliant on the optics of the eye; any media opacities and corneal irregularities will affect the image obtained. In these cases, dilation may well be beneficial to achieve an optical angle between the camera chip and the fundus with minimal disruption. It is also important to note that the image obtained will depend on the refractive error of the patient. The change in image size with refractive error varies between cameras, but has been found to be approximately 5 to 30% (Rudnicka et al 1998, Coleman et al 1996). This should not cause a problem in estimating the cup-to-disc ratio or in estimating size or the position of lesions based on disc diameters, but will affect the accuracy of caliper measurements unless refractive error is taken into account. Even

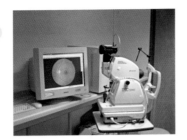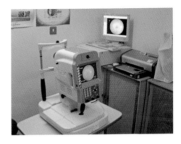

Figure 5.2 Example of a detachable camera (left) and integrated camera (right) fundus imaging system.

then, the ability to monitor a lesion over time will not be affected unless different cameras are used. Some retinal camera systems have a universal attachment (such as a 'C' mount) to their optics so that more than one commercially available camera option can be attached (Fig. 5.2). Commercially available cameras tend to be competitively priced and have the advantage that they can be replaced with newer cameras as technology improves.

Luminance

Once the fundus image has been aligned and focused using the black and white image, image capture is achieved with a colour camera and with the fundus illuminated with a flash (see p. 24). This occurs faster than the pupil can react to prevent a constricted pupil affecting the image. Retinal reflectance varies widely between individuals, presumably due to the pigmentation of the retina and optical transparency of the cornea and crystalline lens, so several images may need to be taken to optimize the image captured. Obviously the fewer images that have to be taken and the lower the flash intensity, the more comfortable the patient. Therefore learning to 'guestimate' the appropriate flash intensity from previous examination (retinoscopy reflex or ophthalmoscopy) and the black and white alignment image is a useful skill. Recording of the flash intensity used on the image not only saves time for subsequent monitoring, but also allows more equivalent images to be taken.

Image manipulation

Complete colour control of the captured image is necessary to be able to highlight important features, such as blood vessels and haemorrhages. Cameras capture raw information regarding the amount of light falling on each pixel location and process this before storing it in a standard image file (usually a TIF image format) on the connected computer or internal media. Single-chip cameras have a red, green or blue colour filter over each pixel and require processing to produce a colour image (see 'Capture technology' section on pp. 11–14). Enhancing blood vessels (and haemorrhages or aneurysms if present) can be achieved by application of a green filter to the image, or by dropping out the red and blue sensitive pixels, leaving the green (Fig. 5.3).

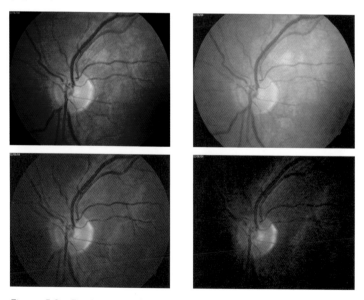

Figure 5.3 Fundus image (top left) split into its red (top right), green (bottom left) and blue (bottom right) components.

As well as altering the colour balance, most imaging programs allow the user to make calibrated measurements of fundus features, magnify the image and enhance the brightness and contrast (with the application of an electronic filter). With the increased interest in diabetic retinopathy screening over the past few years, there have been attempts to automatically detect, highlight and grade retinal features of interest such as haemorrhages (e.g. Sinthanayothin et al 1999, Hipwell et al 2000, Ege et al 2000, Basu et al 2003). As yet there does not appear to be any commercially available software, although much company research and development has been invested in this area and a launch of such software seems imminent. Other useful developments for fundus image viewing have been composite images where a range of images (usually about seven) can be taken with the patient looking in set locations, which are subsequently 'stitched' together using software to give a larger field of view of up to 85° (Fig. 5.4). Some software is capable of displaying stereo image-pairs with the appropriate goggles (captured by imaging the fundus image twice from different locations or angles) and has overlay or comparison functions to enable enhanced image comparison taken on different visits. Many fundus cameras available on the market are also designed to enhance and capture fluorescein angiography.

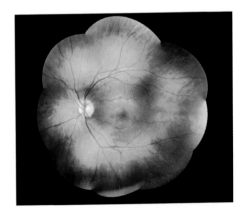

Figure 5.4 Fundus mosaic made up of nine 45° standard images 'stitched' together using registration software.

Resolution and field of view

As explained on page 18, although resolution is often made out to be the principal factor of importance in purchasing an imaging system, it is only one of a number of factors necessary to allow good image capture. The resolution of most standard monitors is only 1280×1024 pixels (1.3 million pixels) and therefore viewing an image taken at a higher resolution than this, without magnification, can potentially lead to slight image degradation (due to the computer having to interpolate the data to the maximum resolution of the screen – Wolffsohn and Peterson 2006). Also by packing more pixels into the same size chip, the light received by any one pixel is reduced, resulting in the need for increased flash luminance/light integration time (reduced shutter speed). This could increase the proportion of ungradable images due to age-related media opacities (estimated in previous studies as between 3.7 and 22% although <5% is achievable with pupil dilation; e.g. Pugh et al 1993). The National Screening Committee has suggested that an acceptable rate of non-gradable images for diabetic screening is 3–5%.

The National Screening Committee has also determined that the minimum pixel resolution required for diabetic screening is 20 pixels per degree (from theoretical consideration of the minimum sized retinal feature of interest) and that no compression of the image should occur (see 'Compression' section on pp. 34–39). However, subsequent research has suggested that compressed JPEG images may be adequate (Basu et al 2003). The original resolution criterion was quoted in terms of lines per millimetre. This equated to 1000×1000 pixels, but as the minimum field of view required is 45° horizontally and 40° vertically, the equivalent pixel resolution requirement of a camera was adjusted to 1365×1000 pixels (assuming the normal round image and approximately 90% usage of the image area; British Diabetic Association 1999). Few newly released retinal cameras fall below this resolution. The Nidek NM200D camera only has a 30° field of view, although this limitation is more than made up for by its portable nature. It is compact, rather than particularly light, having an unconstrained measurement head and a built-in

Figure 5.5 Nidek NM200D portable fundus camera.

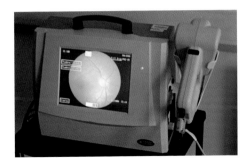

touch-screen monitor/processor, which is ideal for domiciliary visits and providing screening in care homes and for young children (Fig. 5.5). It also has a video output allowing the potential to record an examination of an uncooperative patient in which only a momentary glimpse of the fundus may be achieved.

Fluorescein angiography

Novotny and Alvis described the intravenous use of fluorescein sodium together with retinal photography to examine the integrity of the retinal vasculature in 1961. Fluorescein dye has a peak excitement wavelength of ~490 nm and emits a yellow-green light (~520–530 nm), although this is dependent on the pH of the environment (in this case the blood, which has a pH of ~7.6) and the concentration of the dye. 3–5 ml of 10% fluorescein sodium is injected into a vein in the lower arm or into the antecubital vein in the space below the elbow. The volume of dye injected depends on the height and weight of the patient (body mass index). Smaller volumes of 20–25% solution give better results in eyes with hazy media. Approximately 80% of the dye molecules bind to serum protein on entering the circulating blood, with the remaining unbound fluorescein molecules available to fluoresce when excited with light of the appropriate wavelength. The dye is metabolized by the kidneys and is eliminated through the urine within 24 to 36 hours of administration. The technique is useful in a range of conditions such as macular degeneration, diabetic retinopathy, hypertensive retinopathy and vascular occlusions.

The dye takes ~3–5 seconds to appear in the choroidal circulation following the injection. A series of timed photographs are taken through previously dilated pupils in quick succession to capture the five phases of fluorescein angiography (Danesha 2000):

1. pre-arterial – choroidal circulation fills resulting in choroidal flush
2. arterial
3. capillary (arteriovenous)
4. venous
5. after – leaked dye remains in the retina for about 20 minutes.

Before injecting the dye, the fundus camera focusing and illumination is optimized for the patient under investigation. The time taken for the dye to reach the retina from injection in the arm varies, but is typically 10–12 seconds. The early transit phases (first four) are the most critical part of the angiogram and usually last less than a minute. The image sequence ideally commences just before the dye is visible, at one image each second (1 Hz) until maximum fluorescence occurs. Due to this time demand to image the initial phase, only one eye can be imaged, although photographs of the fellow eye or other areas of interest in the retina can be taken subsequently. Late phase photographs are taken as the dye dissipates, usually 7 to 15 minutes after the injection (Fig. 5.6). Vascular abnormalities lead to hyperfluorescence (dye leaking) or hypofluorescence (areas where blood perfusion is inadequate). Features such as drusen hyperfluoresce as they take in dye, whereas pre-retinal haemorrhage blocks the view of the underlying retina and appears dark. Patients should be warned that the skin and mucous membranes may be stained (pale yellow) for a few hours following the injection and urine (coloured fluorescent green) for up to 2 days. Approximately 10% of patients feel nauseous after the injection, but this typically lasts less than 1 minute and rarely

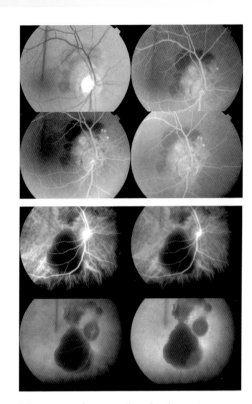

Figure 5.6 The stages of fluorescein (top panel) and indocyanine green (bottom panel) angiography in a patient with idiopathic choroidal vasculopathy after two separate episodes of subretinal haemorrhage (courtesy of Jonathan Gibson FRCS).

leads to vomiting. Although there are no known risks or adverse reactions associated with pregnancy, most practitioners will avoid performing fluorescein angiography in pregnant women, especially in their first trimester (Halperin et al 1990). Nursing mothers should be cautioned that fluorescein is also excreted in human milk (Mattern and Mayer 1990).

Not all fundus cameras enable rapid time recorded sequential photography with optimized blue light and barrier filters (see 'Fluorescein' section on pp. 57–62). Stereo photographs (during portions of the angiogram) can be useful in identifying the histopathological location of angiographic findings within the retina. Fluorescein angiography can also be recorded using a confocal scanning laser ophthalmoscope (see 'Scanning laser ophthalmoscope' section on pp. 92–97), avoiding the need for pupil dilation in some patients.

The wavelength emitted by fluorescein angiography is largely blocked by the retinal pigment epithelium (RPE) and the dye readily diffuses through the choriocapillaris, so it is not well-suited to view the choroidal circulation. Indocyanine green avoids these issues as it fluoresces in the near-infrared (~835 nm), but fluoresces much less than fluorescein. The reduced blocking effect of the RPE, combined with the slower perfusion through the choroidal circulation, makes indocyanine green angiography particularly useful in the examination of choroidal neovascular membranes, such as those that occur in age-related macular degeneration (Fig. 5.6).

As well as intravenous fluorescein, oral fluorescein can be useful in evaluating many retinal conditions characterized by bright late leakage, such as cystoid macular oedema. Fundus photographs taken 40–60 minutes after ingestion of 25 mg/kg of bodyweight provide a good image in ~75% of patients. There are no reports of oral fluorescein causing serious reactions (which occur in ~0.05% of cases with intravenous injection of fluorescein), and minor adverse effects (which occur in up to 20% of cases with intravenous injection of fluorescein) are also uncommon (Watson and Rosen 1990, Kelley and Kincaid 1992). Oral fluorescein angiography, composite images and the use of stereoscopic imaging of the fundus (available on several of the retinal cameras on the market) are some of the features being considered with regard to diabetic screening (Shiba et al 1999, Razvi et al 2001, Rudnisky et al 2002).

Retinal microperimeter

The microperimeter MP-1 is a new 45° fundus camera with an integral computerized fields machine, so that visual light sensitivity

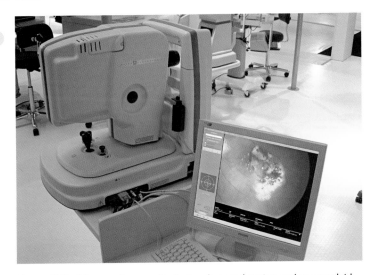

Figure 5.7 Microperimeter displaying damaged retina and an overlaid field plot.

in areas of retinal damage can be examined in detail and the results overlaid (Fig. 5.7). Infrared light allows real-time, non-mydriatic observation of the fundus during visual field assessment together with high speed tracking to ensure true registration of light sensitivity and fundus location. A region of interest can be selected to optimize rapid tracking, making the examination faster and more reliable. The visual field assessment is flexible, allowing the level of automation and parameters such as stimulus size to be set. Fixation during the examination can be displayed as dots overlaid on the image and various analyses are performed.

Scanning laser ophthalmoscopes

Instead of using a pixel matrix to image the fundus, scanning laser ophthalmoscopes measure the reflectance of light at individual successive points on the fundus scanned by a laser in a raster pattern. The results are then formed into an image, much like a conventional cathode ray tube television. As only a single point is imaged at any one time, the light can be much brighter than would be tolerated by conventional photography, often resulting in a more clearly defined image.

Optos Panoramic200

This is a scanning laser ophthalmoscope that uses a wide ellipsoidal mirror to image the retina through an undilated pupil. Collimated low-powered red and green laser beams are deflected in the horizontal and vertical meridians to scan the fundus in 0.25 seconds, producing a high resolution (up to 2000×2000 pixels) digital colour image of virtually the entire retina (200°). The green channel (532 nm laser) image contains information from the sensory retina through to the pigment epithelium layers of the retina. The red channel (633 nm laser) image contains information from the deeper structures of the retina, from the pigment epithelium through to the choroid. Elliptical mirrors have two focal points that are conjugate. The lasers are focused on one focal point on the elliptical mirror and image a second focal point where the eye is located, hence the ability to image a wide field of view (Fig. 5.8). The light from the two lasers, reflected by the retina, is then separated into its red and green components and reassembled into a colour image.

Due to the combination of red and green images of different retinal layers, the fundus pictures look very different to those conventionally seen from standard fundus cameras (see p. 20) capturing red, green and blue light from the retinal surface (Fig. 5.9).

Peripheral retinal lesions, difficult to image with conventional retinal cameras, can be observed using this instrumentation (Fig. 5.10).

Heidelberg Retinal Tomograph (HRT)

This is a confocal scanning laser ophthalmoscope that provides objective quantitative measurements of the optic nerve head and surrounding retinal nerve fibre layer (Fig. 5.11). Retinal damage occurring in glaucoma has traditionally been evaluated with perimetry. However, it has been shown that as many as 40–50%

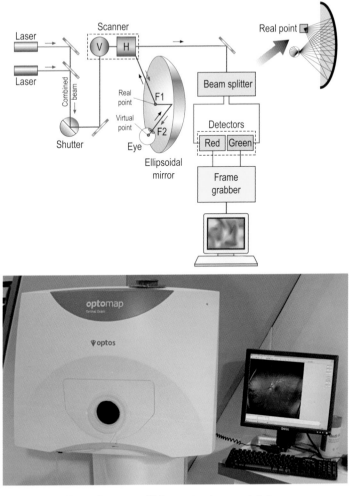

Figure 5.8 Optos Panoramic200 scanning laser ophthalmoscope.

of ganglion cells can be lost before a visual field defect can be detected (Quigley et al 1982, Kerrigan-Baumrind et al 2000). Another limitation of perimetry is the often poor repeatability of this subjective test (Keltner et al 2000).

Clinical research with the HRT has shown that the automated results are comparable or better than expert interpretation of

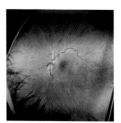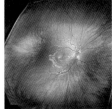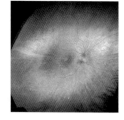

Figure 5.9 Panoramic200 simulated colour (left), green (retinal layers – middle), and red (choroidal layers – right) of a healthy fundus.

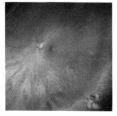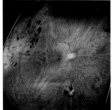

Figure 5.10 Panoramic200 images of cobblestone degeneration (left) and a treated peripheral retinal detachment (right) (courtesy of Optos).

high quality stereo photographs of the optic disc (Zangwill et al 2004, Wollstein et al 2000). HRT measurements have been shown to have high diagnostic accuracy for detecting glaucoma, with a sensitivity and specificity of around 90% (Wollstein et al 1998, Swindale et al 2000, Bowd et al 2002). Reproducibility of the measures is also good (Chauhan et al 1994, Bathija et al 1998, Rohrschneider et al 1994). HRT measurements of structural changes to the cup, rim and retinal nerve fibre layer (RNFL) can detect optic disc abnormalities in glaucoma-suspect eyes several years before the development of visual field defects (Bowd et al 2004, Kamal et al 1999, Tan and Hitchings 2003). This fits well with the new emerging definition of glaucoma as 'progressive structural optic nerve damage'. The software identifies areas of change, qualifies the rate of change and indicates the statistical significance of the change (i.e. whether it is likely to be real rather than due to physiological variability).

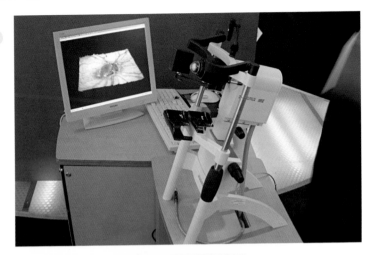

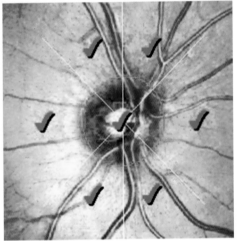

Figure 5.11 Heidelberg Retinal Tomograph (HRT II).

The HRT can also be utilized to examine other areas of the retina, such as the macula in suspected oedema. A Rostock Cornea module can be added to the instrument to create a confocal microscope, allowing single scan movies of up to 30

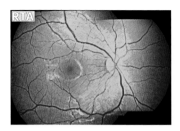 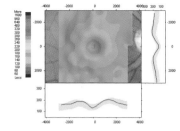

Figure 5.12 Retinal thickness analyser fundus image (left) and disc thickness analysis (right).

frames or volume images of up to 40 frames over 400 μm^2 (384 pixels by 384 pixels).

Retinal thickness analyser (RTA)

The retinal thickness analyser projects a vertical narrow green helium-neon (543 nm) laser slit beam at an angle on the retina while a CCD camera records the backscattered light. Due to the oblique projection of the beam and the transparency of the retina, the backscattered light returns two peaks corresponding to the vitreoretinal and the chorioretinal interfaces. The calculated algorithm distance between the two light peaks determines the retinal thickness at a given point. A 3×3 mm scan consisting of 16 optical cross-sections is acquired within 0.3 seconds. Five such scans are obtained at the macula, three scans at the disc, and additional five scans cover the peripapillary area. During scanning, the RTA acquires a red-free fundus image. Using blood vessels as guidelines, registration software automatically overlays the map on the fundus image, enhancing reproducibility and measurement accuracy (Fig. 5.12). Using edge detection analysis, the topography algorithm identifies the left border of the light, corresponding to the vitreoretinal surface, and calculates the disc topography. In order to obtain quantitative stereometric measurements, the examiner draws a contour line along the disc edge, which is used in follow-up visits to ensure accurate monitoring of subtle changes. Hoffman et al 2005 found a moderate agreement on optic disc parameters between RTA, OCT and HRT II, but there were discrepancies between them. Macular oedema from diabetic retinopathy was more reliably detected with OCT and HRT II than with RTA (Guan et al 2004, Goebel and Franke 2006).

Optical coherence tomography

Optical coherence tomography (OCT) is a non-invasive optical method allowing cross-sectional imaging (pp. 74–77). Its principal application has been in retinal assessment where it has been used to section through the retinal layers, particularly in the macular region, such as in the assessment of macular oedema and macular degeneration (Polito et al 2006, Pieroni et al 2006; Fig. 5.13). The technique shows good inter- and intra-examiner repeatability, but gives lower values for retinal thickness than the retinal thickness analyser described in the preceding section (Krist et al 2005). OCT measures of retinal nerve fibre layer thickness have been shown to be a good independent predictor of the development of glaucomatous change in glaucoma suspects, even when adjusting for stereophotograph assessment, age, intraocular pressure, central corneal thickness and automated perimetry pattern standard deviation (Lalezary et al 2006, Parikh et al 2007). OCT has also been combined with adaptive optics to allow visualization of individual retinal pigment epithelium cells (Roorda et al 2007). Multiple OCT section images can be spatially registered to construct a three-dimensional image (Fig. 5.13). These constructed in-vivo images have been compared to histological examination in animal retinas and shown to correspond well (Ruggeri et al 2007). Quantitative assessments such as volume measures can be determined and followed longitudinally, enhancing the study of ocular disease. Recent instruments are dual-channel systems, combining OCT with scanning laser ophthalmoscopy to enable clinicians to locate areas of interest in standard fundus images and to simultaneously observe a retinal section at this location.

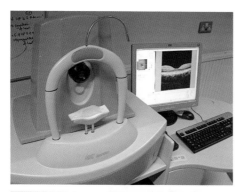

Figure 5.13 Optical coherence tomographer (top) showing a retinal slice (middle) and 3D composite of 50 slices (bottom).

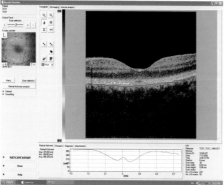

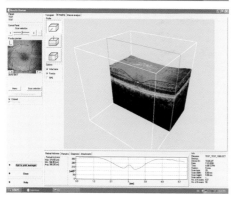

Scanning laser polarimetry (GDx)

The scanning laser polarimeter, the GDx VCC, measures the phase shift (retardation) of polarized light passing through the eye in 0.8 seconds using GaAlA's 780–798 nm laser diode (Fig. 5.14). Retardation is affected by the arrangement and density of RNFL microtubules or other directional elements and tissue thickness. The new variable corneal compensation (VCC) feature determines and corrects for each patient's individual non-RNFL retardation as scanning laser polarimetry measurements can be influenced by several conditions such as corneal birefringence (Zhou and Weinreb 2002). The software compares each patient's RNFL measurements imaged over 20° by 40°, to an age-stratified, multi-ethnic normative database (Fig. 5.15). The GDx VCC nerve fibre index (generated by neural network techniques) allows easy, rapid and accurate discrimination between healthy and primary open angle glaucomatous eyes (Reus and Lemij 2004a, Medeiros et al 2004). GDx VCC measurements of the peripapillary RNFL relate well with functional visual field loss in glaucoma and it has

Figure 5.14 GDx VCC measurement principle and instrument.

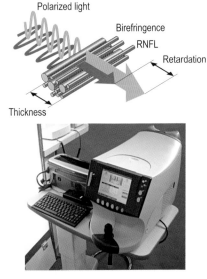

Polarized light

Birefringence

RNFL

Retardation

Thickness

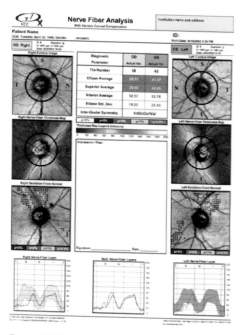

Figure 5.15 GDx VCC nerve fibre analysis data of the right and left eye. On the colour maps, warm colours (such as reds) indicate greater retinal nerve fibre layer values and cooler colours (such as blues) show lower values. The central upper panel gives the nerve fibre index based on a neural network, with higher values (towards 100) indicating greater certainty of glaucoma.

been suggested that the GDx VCC is able to monitor mild glaucoma better than perimetry (Reus and Lemij 2004b, Bagga and Greenfield 2004; Fig. 5.16).

Ultrasonography

Ultrasonography uses high frequency mechanical pulses to assess the biometry of the eye with a 10–20 MHz transducer, achieving a resolution of about 100 μm (see Fig. 4.21). High frequency ultrasound biomicroscopy (UBM) has a tissue penetration depth

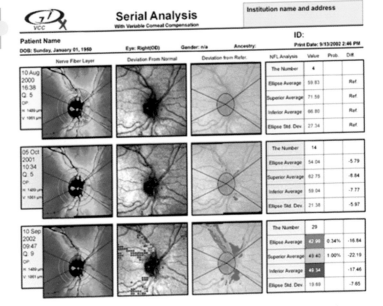

Figure 5.16 GDx VCC nerve fibre analysis serial analysis. This shows the change in retinal nerve fibre layer from the baseline (top) image over time.

of only 4–5 mm, so cannot be used to image the retina (see 'Ultrasonography' section on p. 77).

Computerized tomography

Computerized tomography (CT or CAT) emits several simultaneous X-rays from different angles (see 'Computerized tomography' section on p. 79). For the eye CT scans are usually used to assess ocular trauma, especially if a metal foreign body is suspected in which case MRI is contraindicated (Kolk et al 2005).

Magnetic resonance imaging

Magnetic resonance imaging (MRI) uses electromagnetic waves combined with the reception of weak radio signals to record the density or concentration of hydrogen (or other) nuclei in the body (Charman 1998; see 'Magnetic resonance imaging' section on pp. 79–80). Three-tesla systems are now available, allowing improved imaging of the eyes, and small receiver coils can be used on the ocular surface to create high resolution images of the globe. Three-dimensional models can be constructed from the anatomical slices, for example for the examination of retinal shape with refractive error (Singh et al 2006). Magnetic resonance angiography can be used to assess retinal blood vessels.

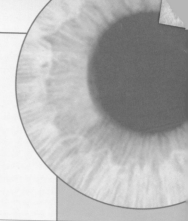

6
Imaging considerations

Tear film

The thin clear tear film is difficult to image. Fluorescein can be instilled to make the tear film more visible, but this is considered an invasive technique as it may affect tear film dynamics (Mengher et al 1985, Johnson and Murphy 2005; pp. 57–62; Fig. 3.1). A 'cold' light source, such as that projected onto the cornea by the Tearscope (Keeler, Fig. 6.1) and most Placido topographers (see pp. 69–71), is thought to have minimal effect on the tear film due to its low intensity and heat output. In addition, the lipid layer thickness can be assessed from the light patterns observed, with thicker tear films showing coloured fringes, average thickness an amorphous pattern and thin films a meshwork pattern. Specular reflection of the first Purkinje image can make the tear film visible, particularly in indirect illumination (see p. 66; Fig. 4.14). Tear break-up time is usually measured subjectively, but dynamic analysis of a Placido disc allows objective measurement (Iskander and Collins 2005). A confocal scanning laser ophthalmoscope has been modified to image the tear film break-up at high (200×) magnification (Torens et al 2000).

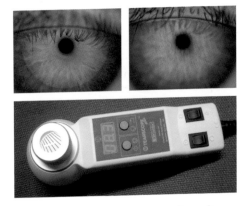

Figure 6.1 Tearscope view of the tear film showing amorphous (top left) and wave (top right) lipid layer patterns.

Cornea

The transparency of the cornea allows the different layers to be imaged using techniques such as slit-lamp and Scheimpflug optic (pp. 63 and 68), confocal microscopy (pp. 73–74) and optical coherence tomography (pp. 74–77). This can quantify the depth of foreign bodies and incisions, corneal thickness and corneal transparency. Total internal reflection of light (sclerotic scatter – pp. 65–66) and back illumination (retro-illumination – p. 65) can be utilized to identify corneal incursions, such as oedema, microcysts and vacuoles. The endothelium is best imaged using slit-lamp specular reflection of the second Purkinje reflection under high magnification, or confocal microscopy. Front surface corneal topography can be assessed by Placido disc or raster scan (pp. 69–72; Fig. 4.18). The back surface curvature of the cornea can be assessed by raster scan and rotating Scheimpflug techniques (p. 68). A red-free (usually green) filter can be used to increase the contrast of neovascularization or scleral and conjunctival blood vessels. Direct and diffuse techniques (pp. 63–64) are generally used to observe surrounding tissue such as the bulbar and palpebral (under the inverted eyelid) conjunctiva. Rotating the diffuse light source to the opposite side of the eye from that being imaged helps to minimize reflections.

Rose bengal and lissamine green

These dyes can be instilled onto the anterior eye to highlight conjunctival damage (diagnostic of dry eye disease; Fig. 6.2), in comparison to fluorescein (pp. 57–62), which is better at

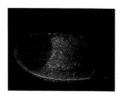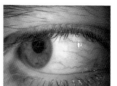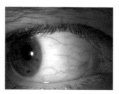

Figure 6.2 An eye stained with fluorescein (left), lissamine green (middle) and rose bengal (right).

highlighting damage to the cornea. Rose bengal uptake is inhibited by albumin, mucin or carboxy cellulosis, so staining occurs when there is insufficient protection of pre-ocular tear film as a result of decreased tear components or abnormal surface epithelial cells (Feenstra and Tseng 1992). Blepharospasm and tearing occurs frequently after application and it has been shown to be toxic to corneal cells, hence it is not really a vital dye (Feenstra and Tseng 1992). Norn introduced lissamine green into ocular examination in 1973. It stains membrane degenerate cells and dead cells in a similar manner to rose bengal, but causes less irritation and toxicity to eyes (Manning et al 1995). It is usually viewed in white light, although in a few reports, a red filter has been employed in the illumination system.

Anterior chamber

The anterior chamber can be imaged in cross-section by techniques such as slit-lamp and Scheimpflug optic section (pp. 63–64 and 68), confocal microscopy (pp. 73–74), optical coherence tomography (pp. 74–77), B-scan ultrasonography (pp. 77–78), computerized tomography (p. 79) and magnetic resonance imaging (pp. 79–80). This can aid visualization of the angle of the corneal iris angle (where the aqueous humour drains through the canal of Schlemm) and iris tumours. A gonioscopy lens can be placed on the cornea, to overcome total internal reflection of light which otherwise obscures the anterior chamber angle, by the use of its lens curvature or angled mirrors (Fig. 6.3). Other techniques, such as the ratio of the corneal thickness to the distance between the endothelium and iris, when an optic section at 60° to the visual axis is positioned at the limbus, can be imaged to assess the anterior chamber depth (Van Herrick's technique – Table 6.1; Fig. 6.4). Inflammation of the uvea, which can occur with eye infection as well as some systemic conditions, can be determined by the presence of cells and flare in the anterior chamber, best imaged with slit-lamp conic beam illumination (pp. 63–64). The edge of the iris should also be examined for synechia with the crystalline lens surface.

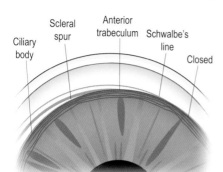

Ciliary body | Scleral spur | Anterior trabeculum | Schwalbe's line | Closed

a

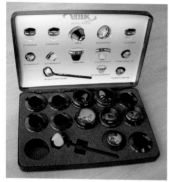

b

Figure 6.3 **(a)** Schematic of the anterior chamber angle view from open (left) to closed (right) conditions. **(b)** A set of gonioscope lenses.

Crystalline lens

Due to its position behind the iris, the crystalline lens is difficult to image without dilation. However, pharmaceutical dilation of the pupil affects ocular accommodation and therefore makes the assessment of changes in crystalline or intraocular lens shape with accommodation difficult to achieve, except for methods such as magnetic resonance imaging (pp. 79–80). The central front surface can be imaged using specular reflection of the third

Table 6.1 **Van Herrick's technique findings and its clinical interpretation**

Grade	Ratio of aqueous gap/cornea	Clinical interpretation
4	>½/1	Closure impossible
3	½–¼/1	Closure impossible
2	¼/1	Closure possible
1	<¼/1	Closure likely with full dilation
0	Nil	Closed

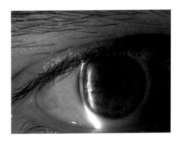

Figure 6.4 Van Herrick's technique on an open anterior chamber.

Purkinje image (p. 66; Fig. 4.14). Optical coherence tomography cannot penetrate the pigmented iris, but can image the lens well through the pupil (pp. 74–77). Scheimpflug (p. 68) and optic section techniques (pp. 63–64) can image the front of the lens though the pupil and give an idea of crystalline lens transparency, but do not allow the posterior lens surface or lens thickness to be assessed. Observation of the lens capsule size, lens fibrosis following phacoemulsification, intraocular lens positioning and the migration of lens epithelial cells to cause posterior capsular opacification will become more important with the development of advanced intraocular lens designs such as those aiming to restore accommodation.

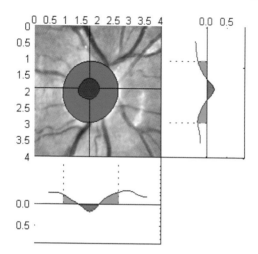

Figure 6.5 Retinal thickness analyser optic disc analysis.

Optic disc

As well as fundus photography (pp. 82–83), the optic disc can be imaged by scanning laser ophthalmoscopy (pp. 92–97), optical coherence tomography (pp. 98–99, Fig. 5.13) and scanning laser polarimetry (pp. 100–101, Figs 5.15 and 5.16). The cup depth, profile and cup-to-disc ratio can be calculated (Fig. 6.5). The disc margin normally needs to be defined subjectively, influencing the results, but can be used in subsequent analysis of the same person. Scanning laser polarimetry assesses the retinal nerve fibre layer in the area surrounding the disc, an important indicator for glaucoma.

Macula

As with the optic disc (p. 111), the macula can be imaged by conventional fundus photography (pp. 82–83), scanning laser ophthalmoscopy (particularly the Heidelberg Retinal Tomograph – pp. 93–97), optical coherence tomography (pp. 98–99) and scanning laser polarimetry (pp. 100–101). The macular thickness, profile and underlying detachments or oedema can be assessed.

Retinal shape

Retinal shape can be assessed by B-scan ultrasonography
(pp. 101–102), computerized tomography (p. 102) and
magnetic resonance imaging (p. 103). Three-dimensional models
can be built up from multiple scans, allowing assessment of the
shape of the globe in conditions such as the development of
myopic refractive error.

Retinal features

Retinal features, such as detachments, peripheral degeneration
and naevi can be imaged by conventional fundus photography
(pp. 82–83; including the microperimeter – pp. 91–92) and
scanning laser ophthalmoscope (pp. 92–97). The Optos
Panoramic200 gives a 200° field of view, allowing the retinal
periphery to be imaged without the need for eye rotation (p. 93;
Figs 5.8–5.10). Most fundus cameras have a method for moving
the fixation target, so the peripheral retina can be examined,
although pupil dilation is usually required to achieve a wide field
of view.

Red-free filter photography has been utilized as
monochromatic illumination can enhance the visibility of various
ocular features, accentuating the difference in reflectance
between the structure and the background; for example, vascular
walls have their optimum visibility between 445 and 510 nm and
vessels, haemorrhages and microaneurysms between 530 and
590 nm yellow/green light (Duerey et al 1979, Weinberger et al
1999). This effect can be best achieved by using the signal from
the green pixels of the CCD/CMOS array alone. It is noteworthy
that the colour sensitivity of a digital camera and the sensitivity
of the human visual system do not correspond exactly and a
filter which gives the best subjective visual observation contrast
may not be the best to use in a digital system (Owen 2000).

There have been attempts to automatically detect, highlight
and grade retinal features of interest such as haemorrhages

(e.g. Sinthanayothin et al 1999, Hipwell et al 2000, Ege et al 2000, Basu et al 2003). Artificial neural networks, which are 'taught' to differentiate diseased retinas from healthy eyes by inputting prediagnosed fundus images, have been applied to conditions such as diabetic retinopathy. Specificity of 88% and sensitivity of 84% compared to the diagnosis of an ophthalmologist have been reported (Gardner et al 1996). It has therefore been estimated that such techniques could reduce the number of patients requiring specialist examination by 70%. However, the sensitivity and specificity of disease detection depends on the quantity, quality and range of image input along with the quality of new images to be analysed.

Retinal grading scales vary in complexity depending on whether they are for clinical or research use, but typically involve up to eight stereo pairs of fundus photographs to cover the areas of interest graded on a 3- to 6-point scale (Diabetic Retinopathy Study Research Group 1981, Klein et al 1984, 1990). Grading of maculopathy has also been established to evaluate the effects of photocoagulation (Early Treatment Diabetic Retinopathy Study Report 1985, Aldington et al 1995).

7
Teleophthalmology

Telecommunication technologies are advancing at an ever increasing pace. These advances are changing the ways in which we live our lives. The specific application of this growing technology to medicine is known as telemedicine. Telemedicine (*telos* from Greek meaning distance and *medicus* from Latin meaning physician) is growing in popularity, especially in remote areas, to allow an expert or second opinion on a medical case. Telemedicine may be defined as a system that electronically transports a consulting physician usually from a hospital setting (host) to a site at a distant (remote) facility where their expertise is required. Telemedicine may be as simple as faxing a copy of a visual field, or as complex as multipoint videoconferencing with high resolution image transfer. The definition of the purposes of telemedicine adopted by the US Congress (House Bill 426, Section 3, introduced in the 104th Congress) was to (1) transmit, compress and archive data; (2) perform examinations and procedures, conduct consultations, and diagnose and treat physical and mental conditions; (3) train health professionals and students; and (4) monitor patients' medical conditions outside a healthcare facility.

The interest in telemedicine has grown steadily, with over 216 projects identified in the UK between 1991 and 2004 (Debnath 2004). It is estimated in the US that over $200 million a year can be saved by the implementation of telemedicine. In the field of ophthalmology, teleophthalmology has mainly been applied to diabetic screening, although in more remote settings such as India, it is being applied to more general ophthalmological diagnosis (Li 1999). Tuulonen and colleagues (1999) tested the feasibility of teleophthalmology applications in examining patients with glaucoma, using a video slit-lamp, an automated perimeter, a non-mydriatic fundus camera and a videoconferencing system installed in a healthcare centre in a rural area linked to a university eye clinic, in comparison to those seen in the university clinic. Both patient groups were equally satisfied with the ophthalmic service. Patients liked the reduction in travelling (97%), costs (92%) and time (92%). The costs of the telemedicine and conventional visits were equal, but decreased travelling saved $55 per visit. However, the quality of the images obtained in the remote centre was poorer than that of the images obtained at the university clinic.

Telemedicine has both social and economic benefits. Social benefits include:

- increased patient access to specialist consultation, enhancing the scope of services provided locally
- easier for friends and relatives to provide support to the patient locally in terms of transportation and visitation (if admitted) than in a distant specialist centre
- decreased geographic isolation of healthcare providers
- improved healthcare provider recruitment and retention in community settings
- improved continuity of care
- enhanced referral relationships
- retention of essential healthcare revenues in rural communities.

Economic benefits include:

- access to patients who would otherwise not receive timely intervention due to the need to travel to a specialist hospital
- savings on transportation costs (both for the patient and health service transportation)
- revenue generated in local communities by keeping a patient admitted rather than transferred to tertiary care facilities
- savings from diagnostic tests duplicated at local and transfer site.

Although these are some of the attractive elements of telemedicine, there are also a number of issues raised by its use.

Transfer of information

The transfer of information and in particular high quality images is a vital aspect of telemedicine. The communication of information between two digital platforms generally occurs via either a digital or analogue link. MODEM (MOdulator-DEModulator) connections, typically using telephone lines, exchange information by first converting digital impulses into analogue tones and then back into digital impulses on the receiving end. In contrast to analogue, digital information is represented by signals encoded as a series of discrete numbers, intervals or steps. ISDN (Integrated Services Digital Network) at 128 kilobits/second gives an average transmission time equivalent to one-fifth of that of most analogue systems.

Security

If patient information is to be passed through the internet, it must be secured from unauthorized viewing and tampering. This is not easy to achieve and it is acknowledged that there will always be hackers, but telemedicine servers should encrypt the information sent (typically 128-bit encryption) and have password protection. An example of this is Danish teleophthalmology, an internet-based system for communication of clinical eye data, freely available for all eye doctors in Denmark. The main function is exchange of clinical eye photos which are encrypted and password protected. DICOM (Digital Imaging and Communication in Medicine) is a standard for putting images via a gateway to a health network along with an American National Standards Institute (ANSI) computer language for this purpose (http://medical.nema.org/).

Remote diagnosis

Remote diagnosis still requires personnel with certain skills in the patient's location to ascertain clinical information from the patient such as visual acuity, intraocular pressures and retinal images. Due to the lack of depth information in a retinal image, many schemes aim for stereoscopic image capture, although the equipment for this is more expensive and more data need to be transmitted back to the advanced assessment centre (host). Some schemes view this assessment in the patient's location as a full consultation, whereas others treat it as just an initial

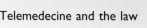

screening with a consultation only taking place if an anomaly is suspected and the patient attends the advanced medical centre. In either case, teleophthalmology has three major advantages.

Firstly, unnecessary referrals are reduced or eliminated. For example, diabetic patients only need to be referred once they have developed proliferative diabetic retinopathy with high risk characteristics, or clinically significant macular oedema. If they have not developed treatable disease, the patient can be followed at a distance without the need to travel to a hospital.

Secondly, following treatment, referred patients can continue to be followed at a distance without the need for further travel. So, for example, having undergone focal laser treatment for clinically significant macular oedema, a patient can then be followed by teleophthalmology at regular intervals, only returning to the hospital if further treatment is required.

Finally, the data collected by teleophthalmology enables a consultant to plan for necessary testing and treatment at the time of a patient's first visit at a specialist centre, saving time and optimizing resources. For example, if a patient is known to have raised intraocular pressures and an enlarged cup-to-disc ratio in advance, a visual field assessment can be scheduled in advance of the appointment with the consultant so that they can view all the relevant clinical data and commence appropriate treatment after discussions with the patient.

These improvements in efficiency decrease the time to treatment as well as the costs to the healthcare system. They also decrease the number of patients travelling to hospitals or advanced medical centres by screening out those who do not need treatment before they attend a hospital.

Telemedecine and the law

Some experts believe telemedicine will lower risks since it usually involves practitioners working together, resulting in more comprehensive patient care. However, in addition to the normal legal issues that relate to any medical consultation, telemedicine has some unique issues relating to the remote nature of the

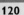

diagnosis and the need to transfer patient information from one location to another.

Medical record ownership and confidentiality   Telemedicine demands that an electronic medical record of the patient be shared. There are issues regarding who will have access to the transmitted information, who is the ultimate custodian of the medical record and who is responsible for ensuring the patient's privacy. In the EU, healthcare data protection standards are being formulated and a 'Euroseal Mark or Certificate' is expected to develop which will 'certify' a healthcare organization as meeting the EU standard for data protection. These issues are further complicated in countries such as the USA, where federal legislation regulating the confidentiality and privacy of data passing over an interstate network is lacking and confidentiality and privacy laws have been enacted on a state or local basis without regard to overlap or consistency across state lines (such as the acceptability of an electronic signature).

> Doctors carry prime responsibility for the protection of information given to them by patients or obtained in confidence about patients. They must therefore take steps to ensure, as far as lies in their control, that the records, manual or computerized, which they keep or which they transmit, are protected by effective security systems with adequate procedures to prevent improper disclosure. (UK General Medical Council Guidance)

The Data Protection Act (implementing the EU Directive) states that:

- Article 25(1): it is illegal to transmit information to another country that does not have adequate data protection laws.
- Article 17: the controller of the data must implement appropriate technical and organizational measures to protect data against accidental or unlawful destruction or accidental loss, alteration, unauthorized disclosure or access and against all other forms of processing. Such measures must ensure a level of security appropriate to the risks represented by the processing and the nature of the data to be protected.

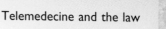

Duty of care   Healthcare systems owe a duty to patients in their facilities to prevent harm negligently caused by them, their employees and agents. As such, they must adequately supervise and credential their staff and independent physicians providing services under their auspices. However, courts have not yet faced the situation where a telemedicine host has no other affiliation with remote physicians and hospitals other than their involvement in the network. The quality of transmitted and stored images must also be adequate for purpose. Failure to have the appropriate equipment, communication failures or adverse incidents involving telemedicine equipment are all new clinical risks involved with telemedicine.

Standards of care   Depending on the relationship between the remote and host specialist centre, the clinical guidelines and standards of care may differ between them. This raises the issue of liability with regard to an appropriate level of care and what happens if the guidelines are not followed.

Negligence issues   It is unclear whether the host or remote facility controls patient care or even the remote practitioners who may ultimately prescribe further diagnosis and treatment based upon the consultation with the host's medical staff.

Consent   Gaining informed consent also becomes an issue when the host consultant never sees the patient and therefore has to rely on a remote centre. Consent to disclosure is required. 'Doctors must give patients the information they ask for or need about their condition, its treatment and prognosis; give information to patients in a way they can understand; [and] respect the right of patients to be fully involved in discussions about care' (HC(90)22 amended by HSG(92)32).

Dispensing of prescriptions   Currently a paper copy of any prescription is required before medications may be dispensed. If the internet is to be legitimately used for dispensing medication, changes in the law will be required.

Jurisdiction   The EU prohibits transporting patients' electronic medical records outside of the EU. In countries such as the USA, hospitals require licensure for their facilities with the state of operation. Therefore if they have a 'virtual' facility in a remote location they provide telemedicine for, they will need additional licences or other assurances of minimum technological standards (such as the minimum resolution of network-transmitted images) from the state of the 'virtual' centre. The same applies to the telephysicians who are now working interstate, particularly if diagnoses and treatment are being applied.

Medical abuse   If doctors are encouraged to refer for second opinions, and get financially rewarded for doing so, there is a risk of unnecessary referrals and accusations of 'kick-back' and fraud. There is also potential for patients to access prescription drugs which had been prohibited by one nation, but available in another or for bogus physicians to dispense medical advice and medications.

Reimbursement   In general, hospitals are funded for the patients they see, so remote services require special financial arrangements between them to fund telemedicine consultations. The use of e-mail has been deemed unprofessional by the British and German Codes of Conduct, and therefore any such interactions are non-reimbursable. Private medical insurance accredits certain medical centres which their members can attend, so telemedicine may require additional remote centres to be accredited in some form. A face-to-face consultation is also normally a requirement for reimbursement. Providers seeking reimbursement must demonstrate medical necessity and this may be more difficult in remote telemedicine consultations.

Laws   Other relevant UK regulations include the EU Data Protection Directive and Act 1998; HSC 1998/153 'Using electronic patient records in hospitals: legal requirements and good practice'; HSG (96)18 'The protection and use of patient information'; HSG(96)15 'NHS information management and technology security manual'; the common law duty of confidentiality; the Computer Misuse Act 1990; Access to Health Records Act 1990; Access to Medical Records Act 1988; and laws relating to public records and electronic documents, and digital signatures.

To get round the medico-legal implications of giving opinion directly to a patient on the internet, as the consultant has not examined the patient themselves, one company offers this service via the patient's general practitioner. Since no patient is sending information to the consultant directly, there is no doctor–patient relationship established. The patient remains under the care of their referring doctor who has the choice of accepting or rejecting the consultant's opinion. Hence it is presumed that current medical malpractice insurance would cover the specialist for giving a second opinion to another physician based on the information provided to them by that physician who has examined the patient, and so protecting the specialist from malpractice suites.

In conclusion, the root cause of the uncertainty about liability related to telemedicine is a lack of relevant legal precedents. Telemedicine technology and practice is still developing and therefore the potential risks are not known, which is problematic for insurance carriers.

Courts will continue applying existing malpractice tests in telemedicine cases, which currently hinge on two key legal questions. Firstly, did a doctor–patient relationship exist? This is not always an easy question to answer. For example, a consultant reviewing a patient's medical records taken by a remote doctor could be interpreted as either an informal consultation between two colleagues or the establishment of a formal physician–patient relationship, depending on the circumstances. The second key legal issue is whether a physician has breached their duty of care. The legal system relies on professional standards to determine appropriate care levels in malpractice cases, and these have not been formulated for telemedicine in most specialties.

Standardization

Due to the great diversity in social, environmental, political and medical systems even within one country, structurally different teleophthalmology programmes may be required to meet local and regional needs. In some countries, such as Canada who have taken much of the lead in teleophthalmology, it has been acknowledged that it is very difficult to be prescriptive in recommendations for prospective teleophthalmology programmes. Nonetheless, efforts should be made to ensure that a degree of internal validation, evaluation, and documentation are part of each telemedicine protocol.

Diagnostic accuracy and reliability

On the whole, teleophthalmology uses less skilled individuals at the initial point of remote contact with the patient than, for example, traditional dilation and fundus examination of diabetics by optometrists. General practitioners in the UK are now financially rewarded for ensuring that their diabetic patients attend one of the local screening centres yearly for fundus photography. This raises the issue of the diagnostic accuracy and reliability of diagnosing diabetic retinopathy that needs treatment using photography rather than a dilated fundus examination. As outlined on pages 87–88, resolution and field of view standards have been placed on diabetic screening photography schemes in the UK and dilation even with the use of non-mydriatic cameras is almost universal. There are still a reasonable proportion of images that are not good enough for grading, mainly due to media opacities, and in these cases a referral to a local optometrist is usually initiated for a dilated slit-lamp biomicroscopy examination.

In general it has been shown that the diagnostic accuracy and reliability of retinal photography is good and the development of computer neural networks to aid the detection of pathological changes should help to increase the efficiency of the detection and subsequent treatment of appropriate pathology. The sensitivity of teleophthalmology for detecting diabetic retinopathy has been shown to be comparable with, if not better than, clinic-based examinations, ranging from 50% to 93%. The specificity of teleophthalmology, like clinic-based examinations, has been consistently high, particularly when both slit-lamp biomicroscopy and stereo fundus examination are involved for the detection of macular oedema (Whited 2006).

In conclusion

Teleophthalmology will continue to develop due to the substantial benefits it can offer. However, the issues surrounding its use will continue to cause concern until they are tested by law, which can only happen with the fullness of time.

Glossary

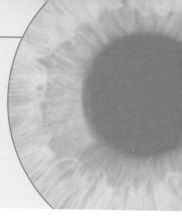

8MM

A common high-end tape format. Current capacities range up to 25 gigabytes.

AD conversion

Analogue–Digital conversion – the conversion of the voltage signal generated by incident light into a binary digital code.

Aliasing

Jagged edges resulting from partial pixel coverage when a line or shape edges are not perfectly horizontal or vertical (staircase effect). Aliasing is less noticeable to the human eye on higher resolution images/displays and can be reduced (known as anti-aliasing) by averaging out the pixels around the edge (both in colour and intensity), making the change more gradual and smooth (blurring effect).

ANSI

A rating for photographic materials devised by the American National Standards Institute.

Aperture

The opening in a camera lens, usually an iris diaphragm, through which light passes to expose the light-sensitive chip or film. Aperture size is usually calibrated in f-numbers. The larger the number, the smaller the lens opening.

Artefact

Undesirable changes to a digital image caused by the sensor, optics and internal image-processing algorithms of the camera.

ASA

American Standards Association – an absolute term indicating a film's sensitivity to light, replaced by ISO (International Organization for Standardization).

ASCII

An acronym for the American Standard Code for Information Interchange; an ANSI binary-coding scheme consisting of 128 seven-bit patterns for printable characters and control of equipment function. ASCII is the basis for information exchange between many computer systems.

Aspect ratio

The ratio of width to height. Used in the imaging industry to define applicability of an image to fit a page, screen, monitor or frame. For example, typically a 35 mm frame is 3:2, a TV is 4:3 and HDTV is 16:9.

Attachment

A file, such as a photograph, sent along with an e-mail message so it can be viewed or saved at the recipient's end.

Autofocus (AF)

Device that focuses the image automatically.

Automatic exposure (AE)

A system that automatically sets correct exposure by linking a camera's exposure meter with the shutter speed or aperture or both.

Bandwidth

General term for the amount of data that can pass through a given channel at one time.

Baud

Named after the French telecommunications technician Baudot. It is the unit used to measure data transfer (1 baud = 1 bit/ second). Therefore, for example, the specification '28 800 bauds' means that data can be transferred at a rate of 28 800 bits per second.

Bayer pattern

A pattern of red, green and blue filters on the image sensor's photosites. There are twice as many green filters as the other colours because the human eye is more sensitive to green and therefore green colour accuracy is more important.

Bayonet lens mount

The most common method of mounting lenses onto a camera body, using a short turn to lock it into place.

Bios

Basic input/output system. The computer part that manages communications between the computer and peripherals.

Bits

Binary digit – the smallest piece of information in a binary numbering system. A binary digit can be either a 0 or 1 and corresponds to one of the millions of 'switches' inside the computer being 'on' or 'off'. Bit depth refers to the greyscale range of an individual pixel. A pixel with 8 bits per colour gives a 24-bit image (8 bits for each of 3 colours is 24 bits).
24-bit colour resolution is 16.7 million colours.
16-bit colour is 65 536 colours.
8-bit is usually 256 shades of grey.

Bitmap

The method of storing information that maps an image pixel, bit by bit. Bitmap file formats include: tiff, bmp and pict.

Blooming

Each pixel (photosite) on a digital camera sensor has a limit as to how much charge it can store. Blooming (or streaking) is the name given to an overflow of charge from an over-saturated pixel (photosite) to the next on the sensor. It can be reduced by gates running beside each row of pixels to allow the overflowing charge to dissipate without affecting surrounding pixels.

bmp

File format extension for bitmap images.

Buffer

A special area set aside either in hardware or software for temporary storage. Usually, the bigger the buffer, the faster the computer can process other data. Buffers allow cameras to take a number of shots in rapid succession without waiting for the previous image(s) to be written to the storage card.

Bus

A path in the computer to transfer information within the computer or to the device(s) to which the data are addressed.

Byte

The standard measurement unit of file size, equal to 8 bits of digital information. 1000 bytes = 1 kilobyte (kB); 1 000 000 bytes = 1 megabyte (MB); 100 000 000 bytes = 1 gigabyte (GB).

Cache

A temporary storage area for information which locates itself between the hard disk and the RAM by employing intuitive logic. It speeds up the access time of the data.

Capacity (storage)

The amount of information, measured in bytes, that can be stored on a device such as a hard drive.

Capture

Acquiring an image by a scanner or digital camera.

Card reader

An electronic device, which is connected to your computer to transfer pictures from memory cards from digital cameras to your computer.

Cathode ray tube (CRT)

The image projection system used in older monitors.

CCD

Charge-Coupled Device, a light-sensitive chip used for image gathering (see p. 9).

Chroma

The quality of a colour that is the combination of hue and brightness. In the Munsell system of colour notation, chroma indicates the purity of a colour as measured along an axis; the farther from the axis, the purer the colour.

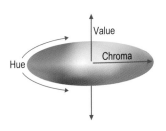

CMOS

Complementary Metal Oxide Semiconductor (see p. 9).

C-mount

A threaded means of mounting a lens to a camera.

CMYK

Cyan, Magenta, Yellow and Key (black). A subtractive colour model, used in colour printing, partly or totally masking certain colours on the typically white background.

Colour balance

The overall hue of the colour in a colour reproduction.

Colour depth

The amount of colour information recorded for each CCD pixel. The greater the depth, expressed in bits, the truer and richer the colour is recorded (see p. 11).

Colour palette

The number of colour shades available for displaying an image.

Colour saturation

The purity of a colour resulting from the absence of black and white.

Colour space

Colour spaces describe how the red, green and blue primaries are mixed to form a given hue in the colour spectrum.

Compact disc (CD)

A storage medium typically capable of holding up to 650 MB of data. CD-R allow data to be recorded on more than one occasion.

CompactFlash

Flash memory card measuring 1.5 inches square, developed by Scandisk. It is used in small portable devices such as digital cameras, MP3 players and PDAs and is available in multiple megabyte capacities.

Compression/Compressed

The re-encoding of data to make it smaller. Some compression schemes maintain the quality of the image (lossless) and some do not (lossy or destructive). Compression speeds processing and transmission time, and reduces storage requirements (see p. 34).

Connectivity

Defines how a camera can be connected to other devices for either the transfer of images or remote control of the camera (see p. 16).

Contrast

The difference in brightness between the lightest and darkest parts of an image.

Conversion

To convert one file format to another.

CPU

Central Processing Unit. A large chip which holds the processing power of the computer.

Crop/Cropping

To trim the edges of an image, to change the composition.

DAT (digital audio tape)

A magnetic tape originally designed for use in audio applications, but now popular for storing back-up data.

Database

A collection of data that is organized so that its contents can easily be accessed, managed and updated.

Default

The setting in a computer program which will take effect if no changes are made.

Definition

Sharpness of an image.

Depth of field/focus

The zone of acceptable sharpness in a picture, extending in front of and behind the plane of the subject, that is most precisely focused by the lens. It is controlled by the size of the aperture (increases with smaller aperture), the distance of the camera from the subject (the further the distance, the greater it is), and the focal length of the lens (greater for a wide angle lens). The depth of focus depends on the f-number of the lens and the acceptable level of blur of an individual.

Device driver

Software that tells the computer how to communicate with a peripheral device, such as a camera or printer.

Diffuser

A filter that spreads light.

Digital

A system which represents information by binary digits (bits). Bits can store a 0 or 1, which can be easily processed and do not suffer from the degradation and noise problems prevalent in analogue circuits.

Digital camera

Instead of using film, digital cameras records data in pixels, representing the light intensity falling on a small square of silicon.

Digital imaging

The recording of light information in the form of binary digits.

Digital zoom

The image is magnified by spacing out the pixels electronically, degrading image quality above the resolution of the eye.

Digitizing

To convert an image into binary code.

Dots per inch (dpi)

The number of pixels per inch on a display device, such as a printer. It is a measure of an output device's resolution and quality.

Download

The process of receiving data from another digital source.

DVD

Digital Video Disc — an optical storage medium that can store up to 4.7 gigabytes (single layer) or up to 17 gigabytes (double sided, double layer).

Dynamic sensor range

The dynamic range of a sensor is defined by the largest possible signal (full well capacity of a pixel) divided by the smallest possible signal (no light exposure or noise floor) it can generate.

Encryption

A technique used in preventing unauthorized third parties from viewing information that you are uploading or downloading. Encryption involves the data being sent being split into sections with each section sent through different connections. The two most common encryption patterns are 56-bit and 128-bit (the higher the number, the more secure the connection is).

Enhancement

The improvement of an image by digital manipulation.

Equalization

An image processing technique where the range of tones or colours in an image file is expanded in order to produce a more pleasing image.

Erase

The process of removing information from memory or storage.

Exif

Exchangeable image file – image file containing additional metadata such as the time and date it was taken and the camera settings.

Export

The process of transporting data from one computer, type of file format, or device to another.

Exposure

The amount of light that passes through a camera lens to form an image. This is dependent on both the aperture and shutter speed and can be optimized using an exposure meter

File format

The way a graphic file is saved, such as TIFF and JPEG (see p. 35).

File size

The amount of computer storage space a file requires, usually measured in kilobytes or megabytes. The file size of an image is proportional to its resolution and the compression applied.

Filter

The use of a coloured medium that selectively absorbs some of the wavelengths of light passing through it to modify the wavelengths of light reaching a light-sensitive material.

FireWire

A very fast external bus that supports data transfer rates of up to 400 megabits per second, developed by Apple.

Flash memory

A memory chip that has the ability to retain image data even after the host system has been shut off.

f-Number (f-stop)

The focal length of a lens divided by its diameter. A sequence of f-numbers calibrates the aperture in regular steps (known as stops) between the minimum and maximum openings of the lens. The f-numbers generally follow a standard sequence, so that the interval between one full stop and the next represents halving or doubling in the image brightness. The f-number becomes progressively higher as the aperture is reduced to allow in less light, i.e. f/5.6, f/8, f/11, f/16, f/22, f/32 . . . Theoretically, all lenses at the same f-number produce images of equal brightness.

Focal length

The distance, usually given in millimetres, between the optical centre of a lens and the point at which rays of light from objects at infinity are brought to focus. In general, the greater the focal length, the smaller and more magnified the part of the scene it includes in the picture frame.

Focus

Position in which rays of light from a lens converge to form a sharp image.

Formatting

Completely erasing and resetting a memory card or disk.

Gain

A method of adjusting a CCD sensor's sensitivity to light to affect the contrast of an image by altering the intensity range.

Gamma

The contrast affecting the mid-level greys or midtones of an image. Each pixel in a digital image has a certain level of brightness ranging from black (0.0) to white (1.0). The gamma describes the relationship (output = input^{gamma}) of how these intensities are displayed on the monitor, where a gamma of 1.0 would respond in a linear way. Due to technical limitations, a CRT typically has a gamma of ~2.5 and an LCD ~2.2. Adjusting the gamma of an image allows you to change brightness values of the middle range of grey tones without dramatically altering the shadows and highlights.

Gamut

The range of colours and tones a device or colour space is capable of recording or reproducing.

Gaussian blur

An image-softening effect utilizing a bell-shaped gaussian distribution.

GIF

A lossless image file format using LZW (Lempel–Ziv–Welch) compression, which is commonly used on the web.

Gigabyte

A measure of computer memory or disk space consisting of one thousand million bytes (a thousand megabytes).

Greyscale

An image type that includes shades of grey assigned to each pixel, typically 8 bits reproducing up to 256 shades.

HSL

Hue, Saturation and Lightness. A method of describing any colour as a triplet of values. The hue represents the colour (wavelength) and is calibrated in degrees about a standard colour wheel. Saturation is the depth of the colour, with 0.0 indicating full grey and 1.0 pure hue (no greyness). The lightness is how black (0.0) or white (1.0) a colour is. A lightness of 0.5 is pure hue.

HTML

HyperText Markup Language. An encoding format for identifying and linking electronic documents used to deliver information on the World Wide Web.

Hue

The aspect of colour that distinguishes it from another colour.

Image capture

The use of a device, such as a scanner or digital camera, to create a digital representation of an image. This digital representation can then be stored and manipulated on a computer.

Image processing

The manipulation of an image to optimize it for viewing.

Image resolution

The amount of data stored in an image file, measured in pixels per inch (dpi).

Image sensor

The type of device used in digital cameras and camcorders to capture an image, such as CCD (charge-coupled device) and CMOS (complementary metal oxide semiconductor). See Chapter 2, page 9.

Intensity

The relative brightness of a portion of the image or illumination source.

Interpolation/Interpolate

To estimate a missing value by taking an average of known values at neighbouring points.

Inverse square law

A law of physics that states that light from a point source decreases inversely to the square of the distance.

ISO

Although the letters actually denote the International Organization for Standardization, they also indicate a film's sensitivity to light (often referred to as its speed). The original term was ASA (American Standards Association). A slow film (ISO rating of ≤100) would need a longer exposure in dim light than would a fast film (ISO ≥400).

JPEG

A graphic file developed by the Joint Photographic Experts Group, involving lossy compression (the amount can be varied). See page 36.

Kernel size

The number of pixels sampled as a unit during image manipulation and sharpening processes.

Kilobyte (kB)

An amount of computer memory, disk space or document size consisting of approximately one thousand bytes. Actual value is 1024 bytes as bits are binary (see Bits on p. 130 and Byte on p. 131).

Lag time

The delay from pressing the shutter release to the camera actually taking the shot. This delay varies between camera models, but is generally decreasing.

LAN

Local Area Network – a communication network that is physically connected by cables, enabling a group of computers to exchange files and share peripherals.

LCD screen

Liquid Crystal Display screen – a monitor which can be used for displaying images and interfacing with camera controls. Different types exist such as TFT (thin film transistor) and DSTN (double super twisted nemantic).

Lens aperture (f/)

The physical opening of a lens. The smaller the f/number, the more light passes through.

Luminance

Lightness of an image.

LUT

Look-Up Table – the table of colours which a computer uses to approximate the desired colour from the range it has available.

Lux

A measurement of the light intensity, equivalent to candle light; 1 lux is equal to 10.76 footcandles.

Macro lens

A lens specially designed to give accurate resolution and a sharp image of a very near subject.

Matrix metering

A matrix metering option uses multiple areas of the frame to calculate the best overall exposure value; available in most digital cameras.

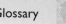

Megabyte (MB)

An amount of computer memory, disk space or document size consisting of approximately one thousand kilobytes. Actual value is 1024 kilobytes as bits are binary (see Bits on p. 130 and Byte on p. 131).

Megapixels

One million pixels or more.

Memory cards

Small memory modules that can be inserted into the camera to hold images, which they retain when power is removed.

Metadata

Information known about the image in order to provide access to the image, such as the intellectual content of the image, digital representation data, and security or rights management information.

Metafile

Files that can be shared by more than one application program.

MHz (megahertz)

A unit of measure for frequency that can relate to the processing speed of a computer. Equal to one million hertz.

Monochrome

Single-coloured. Usually used to describe black and white images.

MPEG

Motion Pictures Expert Group. A motion picture compression system.

Noise

The visible effects of an electronic error (or interference) in the final image from a digital camera. It is affected by temperature (high worse, low better) and sensitivity (high worse, low better).

Optical zoom

Enlarges a subject using a lens (combination of lenses) of variable focal length, without disturbing focus. Unlike digital zoom which only changes the presentation of existing data, the optical zoom actually augments the data collected by the light sensor.

PDF

Portable Document Format – a file format created by Adobe that captures all the elements of a printed document as an electronic image that you can view, navigate, print or forward. PDF files are especially useful for documents in which you want to preserve the original graphic appearance online.

Peripheral

A term used to collectively describe computer accessories such as printers, modems, scanners and external drives.

PICT

A storage format for digital images designed for the Macintosh.

Pixel

Abbreviation of 'picture element', a pixel is a single point in a graphic image. Graphics monitors display pictures by dividing the display screen into thousands or millions of pixels, arranged in rows and columns. The pixels are so close together that they appear connected. The number of bits used to represent each pixel determines how many colours or shades of grey can be displayed. For example, in 8-bit colour mode, the colour monitor uses 8 bits for each pixel, making it possible to display 2 to the 8th power (256) different colours or shades of grey. On colour monitors, each pixel is actually composed of three dots (a red, a blue and a green one). The bit depth and surface size of the individual pixels on an image sensor controls its sensitivity to light (equivalent ISO).

Pixelization

The stair-stepped appearance of a curved or angled line in digital imaging in which the pixel size is large.

Plasma display

A display screen that has gas contained between two panels. When a specified dot is electrically charged, the gas in that area glows.

Plug and play

The ability to install equipment with little or no set-up.

PNG

Portable Network Graphics image format developed as a patent-free alternative to GIF. Provides lossless compression and supports 24-bit images.

Ports

Plugs or connectors into which cables are attached.

PPI

Pixels Per Inch.

Progressive scan

A non-interlaced refresh system for monitors that cuts down on CRT flicker.

RAM

Random Access Memory. The high speed portion of the computer's memory that is held on special chips.

Raster

The series of lines of information such as the parallel and horizontal scan lines that form a television or video display image.

RAW image format

The raw data as it comes directly off the CCD before any in-camera or external processing is performed, making it a true 'digital negative'. It is lossless yet considerably smaller than TIFF and records data over a wider bit range (typically 10 or 12 bits) than JPEG or 8-bit TIFF. However, there is no universally accepted RAW standard format; each manufacturer (even each camera) differs. See page 36.

Reflex camera

A camera that utilizes a mirror system to reflect the light, and therefore the image, coming through the lens, to a visible screen. The image seen in the cameras viewfinder is then the same image entering the lens, providing the most accurate framing and focusing.

Refresh rate

The rate at which an image is redrawn. The faster the refresh rate, the more stable an image will appear and the smoother any movement of the image will be seen.

Resolution

Refers to the sharpness and clarity of an image. The higher the resolution the finer the image detail that can be seen. For printing it is described as the number of dots per inch (e.g. 200 dpi = 40 000 dots printed in a square inch), whereas for graphics monitors and cameras, the resolution signifies the number of dots (pixels) on the entire screen or imaging chip (e.g. 1024 × 768 pixel screen is capable of displaying 1024 distinct dots on each of 768 lines, or 786 432 pixels). This translates into different dpi measurements depending on the size of the screen. VGA resolution is 640 × 480, SVGA 800 × 600, XGA 1024 × 768, and UXGA is used for 1280 × 1024 and 1600 × 1200.

Saturation

The vividness or purity of a colour. The less grey a colour contains, the more saturated it is.

Scanner

A device that captures an image and converts it to a digital form that a computer can display, edit, store and output.

SCSI

A high-speed input/output bus used mainly in Macintosh computers and high-end PCs.

Sepia

A brownish coloured, old-fashioned look to an image often created as a special effect either within a digital camera or in image-editing software.

Serial interface (RS232C or RS422 interface)

An interface which allows peripheral devices such as a mouse, modem and certain digital cameras to be connected to the computer. Data are transferred serially, which means bit by bit, one piece after another, via a connection cable. The serial port is being replaced by the much faster USB port on digital cameras as well as computers.

Server

One computer that acts as a networking device for many interconnected computers.

Sharpening

Electronically enhancing the visibility of a boundary between light and dark tones in an image, resulting in the enhancement of edge detail. It is performed by a mathematical formula which is applied across the image or in a selected region. Most consumer digital cameras apply some level of sharpening as a part of their normal image processing to counteract the effects of the interpolation of colours during the colour filter array decoding process. This can lead to pixelation and other artefacts and is avoided by working from the RAW image format.

Shutter

A movable cover in a camera that controls the time during which light reaches the film. The shutter speed indicates the duration that the shutter is held open during an exposure, which typically ranges from 1/1000th to 1 second. Combined with the lens aperture it controls the total light exposure to the imaging sensor.

Silver halide

A chemical compound of silver (usually silver bromide, silver chloride and silver iodide) used as the light-sensitive constituent (emulsion) in films. The invisible image produced when the halides are exposed to light is converted to metallic silver when the film is subsequently developed.

Smoothing

Averaging pixels with their neighbours to reduce contrast and create an out-of-focus, less pixelated image.

Storage cards

Removable storage device which holds data such as images taken with the camera, such as Compact Flash and Smart Media.

Tagged

An image containing an embedded profile.

Thresholding

When converting a pixel from greyscale to black and white, the threshold is the grey value above which it will be considered white, and below or equal to which it will be considered black.

Thumbnail

A small, low resolution version of a larger image file that is used for quick identification and can allow deletion and protection control.

TIFF

Tagged Image File Format – universal lossless bitmap image used to exchange files between applications and computer platforms.

Transfer rate

The rate at which data can be transferred, usually expressed as kilobits per second (kbps or kbits/s).

TWAIN

Protocol for exchanging information between application and devices such as scanners and digital cameras.

URL

Uniform Resource Locator – a standard addressing scheme used to locate or reference files on the internet. The syntax used is: Scheme://host.domain;port/path filename.

USB

Universal Serial Bus – a plug and play peripheral connection providing power as well as a data transfer stream ~10 times faster than a serial connection.

Vector graphic

A graphic file where an image is represented by continuous functions shapes, as opposed to an image file which is represented by dots (pixels). Vector graphics require less space and can generate much higher quality output which is resizable without a loss in resolution, but work better with less complex electronic art than with real images.

Vignetting

A fall-off in illumination at the edges of an image, usually caused by a lens hood or similar attachment partially blocking the field of view of the lens. It also refers to a printing technique where the edges of the picture are gradually faded out to black or white.

Virtual memory

Disk space on a hard drive that is identified as RAM through the operating system, or other software, used to increase the operating speed of an application.

Virus

A computer program that automatically duplicates itself, usually resulting in the damage or destruction of software and/or data.

White balance

The process by which a camera tries to emulate the human brain to compensate for the perceived colour of an object being affected by the colour of the lighting under which it is viewed. The colour balance assumes that under normal conditions, if a white object can be made to look white, then the remaining colours will be accurate too. If the original lighting is not close to the proper colour temperature (typically daylight), the 'white balance' may reproduce white at the expense of other hues. Most digital cameras feature automatic white balance, such that the camera calculates the best-fit white balance from the overall colour of the image. However, these systems can be fooled, especially if taking a photograph dominated by one colour. A 'white preset' allows measurement from a white object prior to image capture, which the camera will then use (the recorded 'temperature') to correct the subsequent images.

Zip

To compress a file or files into one file. Commonly used to reduce the size of a file to speed up transmission.

Zooming

Enlarging a portion of an image in order to examine detail.

References

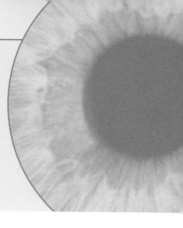

Aldington S J, Kohner E M, Meuer S, et al 1995 Methodology for retinal photography and assessment of diabetic retinopathy: the EURO-DIAB IDDM complications study. Diabetologia 38:437–444

AlSabti K, Raizada S, Wani V B, et al 2003 Efficacy and reliability of fundus digital camera as a screening tool for diabetic retinopathy in Kuwait. J Diabetes Complications 17:229–233

Aslam T M, Patton N, MacGillivray T 2006 The Matrix – image processing, analysis and machine vision in ophthalmology. EyeNews Dec/Jan: 25–30

Atchison D A, Jones C E, Schmid K L, et al 2004 Eye shape in emmetropia and myopia. Invest Ophthalmol Vis Sci 45:3380–3386

Bagga H, Greenfield D S 2004 Quantitative assessment of structural damage in eyes with localized visual field abnormalities. Am J Ophthalmol 137:797–805

Baikoff G, Lutun E, Ferraz C, Wei J 2005 Analysis of the eye's anterior segment with optical coherence tomography. Static and dynamic study. J Fr Ophthalmol 28:343–352

Bailey I L, Bullimore M A, Raasch T W, Taylor H R 1991 Clinical grading and the effects of scaling. Invest Ophthalmol Vis Sci 32:422–432

Basu A, Kamal A D, Illahi W, et al 2003 Is digital image compression acceptable within diabetic retinopathy screening? Diabet Med 20:766–771

Bathija R, Zangwill L, Berry C C, et al 1998 Detection of early glaucomatous structural damage with confocal laser scanning tomography. J Glaucoma 7:121–127

Ben Simon G J, Annunziata C C, Fink J, et al 2005 Rethinking orbital imaging – establishing guidelines for interpreting orbital imaging studies and evaluating their predictive value in patients with orbital tumors. Ophthalmology 112:2196–2207

Bohnke M, Masters B R 1999 Confocal microscopy of the cornea. Prog Ret Eye Res 18:553–628

Bowd C, Chan K, Zangwill L M, et al 2002 Comparing neural networks and linear discriminant functions for glaucoma detection using confocal scanning laser ophthalmoscopy of the optic disc. Invest Ophthalmol Vis Sci 43:3444–3454

Bowd C, Zangwill L M, Medeiros F A, et al 2004 Confocal scanning laser ophthalmoscopy classifiers and stereophotograph evaluation for prediction of visual field abnormalities in glaucoma-suspect eyes. Invest Ophthalmol Vis Sci 45:2255–2262

British Diabetic Association 1999 Guidelines on screening for diabetic retinopathy. London

Bursell S E, Cavallerano J D, Cavallerano A A, et al and the Joslin Vision Network Research Team 2001 Stereo nonmydriatic digital-video colour retinal imaging compared with Early Treatment Diabetic Retinopathy Study seven standard field 35 mm stereo colour photos for determining level of diabetic retinopathy. Ophthalmology 108:572–585

Calkins J L, Hochheimer B F, D'Anna S A 1980 Potential hazards from specific ophthalmic devices. Vision Res 20:1039–1053

Cavanagh H D, El-Agha M S, Petroll W M, Jester J V 2000 Specular microscopy, confocal microscopy, and ultrasound biomicroscopy – diagnostic tools of the past quarter century. Cornea 19:712–722

Charman W N 1998 Imaging in the 21st century. Ophthalmic Physiol Opt 18:210–223

Chauhan B C, LeBlanc R P, McCormick T A, Rogers J B 1994 Test–retest variability of topographic measurements with confocal scanning laser tomography in patients with glaucoma and control subjects. Am J Ophthalmol 118:9–15

Chen T C, Cense B, Pierce M C, et al 2005 Spectral domain optical coherence tomography – ultra-high speed, ultra-high resolution ophthalmic imaging. Arch Ophthalmol 123, 1715–1720

Choma M A, Sarunic M V, Yang C H, Izatt J A 2003 Sensitivity advantage of swept source and Fourier domain optical coherence tomography. Opt Express 11:2183–2189

Coleman A L, Haller J A, Quigley H A 1996 Determination of the real size of fundus objects from fundus photographs. J Glaucoma 5:433–435

Costa M F M, Franco S 1998 Improving the contact lens fitting evaluation by the application of image processing techniques. Int Contact Lens Clin 25:22–27

Cox I 1995 Digital imaging in the contact lens practice. Int Contact Lens Clin 22:62–66

Danesha U 2000 Application of fundus photography in diabetic retinopathy. In: Rudnicka A R, Birch J (eds) Diabetic Eye Disease: Identification and Co-management. Butterworth-Heinemann, Oxford, p 107–112

Debnath D 2004 Activity analysis of telemedicine in the UK. Postgrad Med J 80:335–338

Deramo V A, Shah G K, Baumal C R, et al 1998 The role of ultrasound biomicroscopy in ocular trauma. Trans Am Ophthalmol Soc 96:355–365

Diabetic Retinopathy Study Research Group 1981 Report No. 7. A modification of the Airlie House classification of diabetic retinopathy. Invest Ophthalmol Vis Sci 21:210–226

Dubbelman M, Van der Heijde G L, Weeber H A, Vrensen G F J M 2003 Changes in the internal structure of the human crystalline lens with age and accommodation. Vision Res 43:2363–2375

Duerey N M, Delori F C, Gragoudas E S 1979 Monochromatic ophthalmoscopy and fundus photography. Arch Ophthalmol 97:288–293

Early Treatment Diabetic Retinopathy Study Report 1985 Report No. 1. Photocoagulation for diabetic macular oedema. Arch Ophthalmol 103:1796–1806

Efron N 1998 Grading scales for contact lens complications. Ophthalmic Physiol Opt 18:182–186

Efron N, Morgan P B, Katsara S S 2001 Validation of grading scales for contact lens complications. Ophthalmic Physiol Opt 21:17–29

Efron N, Morgan P B, Jagpal R 2003 The combined influence of knowledge, training and experience when grading contact lens complications. Ophthalmic Physiol Opt 23:79–85

Ege B M, Hejlesen O K, Larsen O V, et al 2000 Screening for diabetic retinopathy using computer based image analysis and statistical classification. Comput Methods Programs Biomed 62:165–175

Feenstra R P G, Tseng S C G 1992 What is actually stained by Rose-Bengal? Arch Ophthalmol 110:984–993

Feng Y W, Simpson T L 2005 Comparison of human central cornea and limbus in vivo using optical coherence tomography. Optom Vis Sci 82:416–419

Fieguth P, Simpson T L 2002 Automated measurement of bulbar redness. Invest Ophthalmol Vis Sci 43:340–347

Fransen S R, Leonard-Martin T C, Feuer W J, Hildebrand P L and the Inoveon Health Research Group 2002 Clinical evaluation of patients with diabetic retinopathy. Ophthalmology 109:595–601

Freegard T J 1997 The physical basis of transparency of the normal cornea. Eye 11:465–471

Freeman G, Pesudovs K 2005 The impact of cataract severity on measurement acquisition with the IOLMaster. Acta Ophthalmol Scand 83:439–442

Friedman D S, Duncan D D, Munoz B, et al 1999 Digital image capture and automated analysis of posterior capsular opacification. Invest Ophthalmol Vis Sci 40:1715–1726

Garcia J A, Fdez-Valdivia J, Fdez-Vidal X R, Rodriguez-Sanchez R 2003 On the concept of best achievable compression ratio for lossy image coding. Pattern Recognition 36:2377–2394

Gardner G G, Keating D, Williamson T H, Elliott A T 1996 Automatic detection of diabetic retinopathy using an artificial neural network: a screening tool. Br J Ophthalmol 80:940–944

Gatinel D, Haouat M, Hoang-Xuan T 2002 A review of mathematical descriptors of corneal asphericity. J Fr Ophtalmol 25:81–90

Goebel W, Franke R 2006 Retinal thickness in diabetic retinopathy – comparison of optical coherence tomography, the retinal thickness analyzer, and fundus photography. Retina 26(1):49–57

Guan K, Hudson C, Flanagan G 2004 Comparison of Heidelberg Retina Tomograph II and retinal thickness analyzer in the assessment of diabetic macular edema. Invest Ophthalmol Vis Sci 45:610–616

Halperin L S, Olk R J, Soubrane G, Coscas G 1990 Safety of fluorescein angiography during pregnancy. Am J Ophthalmol 109:563–566

Hammack G G 1995 Updated video equipment recommendations for slit-lamp videography for 1995. Int Contact Lens Clin 22:54–61

Hashemi H, Yazdani K, Mehravaran S, Fotouhi A 2005 Anterior chamber depth measurement with A-scan ultrasonography, Orbscan II, and IOLMaster. Optom Vis Sci 82:900–904

Hipwell J H, Strachan F, Olson J A, et al 2000 Automated detection of microaneurysms in digital red-free photographs: a diabetic retinopathy screening tool. Diabet Med 17:588–594

Hirano K, Ito Y, Suzuki T, Kojima T, et al 2001 Optical coherence tomography for the noninvasive evaluation of the cornea. Cornea 20:281–289

Hockwin O, Lerman S, Ohrloff C 1984 Investigations on lens transparency and its disturbances by microdensitometric analyses of Scheimpflug photographs. Curr Eye Res 3:15–22

Hoerauf H, Scholz C, Koch P, et al 2002 Transscleral optical coherence tomography – a new imaging method for the anterior segment of the eye. Arch Ophthalmol 120:816–819

Hoffmann E M, Bowd C, Medeiros F A, et al 2005 Agreement among 3 optical imaging methods for the assessment of optic disc topography. Ophthalmology 112:2149–2156

Hom M M, Bruce A S 1998 Image-editing techniques for anterior segment and contact lenses. Int Contact Lens Clin 25:46–49

Iskander D R, Collins M J 2005 Applications of high-speed videokeratoscopy. Clin Exp Optom 88:223–231

Jensen P, Scherfig E 1999 Resolution of retinal digital colour images. Acta Ophthalmol Scand 5:526–529

Johnson M E, Murphy P J 2005 The effect of instilled fluorescein solution volume on the values and repeatability of TBUT measurements. Cornea 24:811–817

Jones C E, Atchison D A, Meder R, Pope J M 2005 Refractive index distribution and optical properties of the isolated human lens measured using magnetic resonance imaging (MRI). Vis Res 45:2352–2366

Kamal D S, Viswanathan A C, Garway-Heath D F, et al 1999 Detection of optic disc change with the Heidelberg Retina Tomograph before confirmed visual field change in ocular hypertensives converting to early glaucoma. Br J Ophthalmol 83:290–294

Keay L, Jalbert I, Sweeney D F, Holden B A 2001 Microcysts: clinical significance and differential diagnosis. Optometry 72:452–460

Kelley J S, Kincaid M 1992 Retinal fluorography using oral fluorescein. Vestn Oftalmol 108:33–34

Keltner J L, Johnson C A, Quigg J M, et al 2000 Confirmation of visual field abnormalities in the Ocular Hypertension Treatment Study. Ocular Hypertension Treatment Study Group. Arch Ophthalmol 118(9):1187–1194

Kerrigan-Baumrind L A, Quigley H A, Pease M E, et al 2000 Number of ganglion cells in glaucoma eyes compared with threshold visual field tests in the same persons. Invest Ophthalmol Vis Sci 41:741–748

King-Smith P E, Fink B A, Fogt N, et al 2000 The thickness of the human precorneal tear film: evidence from reflection spectra. Invest Ophthalmol Vis Sci 41:3348–3359

Klein B E K, Davis M D, Segal P, et al 1984 Diabetic retinopathy: assessment of severity and progression. Ophthalmoscopy 91:10–17

Klein R, Klein B E K, Moss S E 1990 The Wisconsin Epidemiologic Study of diabetic retinopathy; an update. Aus NZ J Ophthalmol 18:19–22

Kocsis O, Costaridou L, Mandellos G, et al 2003 Compression assessment based on medical image quality concepts using computer-generated test images. Comput Methods Programs Biomed 71:105–115

Kolk A, Pautke C, Wiener E, et al 2005 A novel high-resolution magnetic resonance imaging microscopy coil as an alternative to the multislice computed tomography in postoperative imaging of orbital fractures and computer-based volume measurement. J Oral Maxillofac Surg 63:492–498

Koretz J F, Strenk S A, Strenk L M, Semmlow J L 2004 Scheimpflug and high-resolution magnetic resonance imaging of the anterior segment: a comparative study. J Opt Soc Am A 21:346–354

Krist R, Hoffmann E M, Schwenn O 2005 Reproducibility of measurements of the peripapillary retinal nerve fibre layer thickness. Optical coherence tomography versus retinal thickness analyzer. Ophthalmologe 102:1175–1180

Lachenmayr B J, Kojetinsky S, Ostermaier N, et al 1994 The different effects of aging on normal sensitivity in flicker and light-sense perimetry. Invest Ophthalmol Vis Sci 35:2741–2748

Lackner B, Schmidinger G, Pieh S, et al 2005 Repeatability and reproducibility of central corneal thickness measurement with Pentacam, Orbscan, and ultrasound. Optom Vis Sci 82:892–899

Lalezary M, Medeiros F A, Weinreb R N, et al 2006 Baseline optical coherence tomography predicts the development of glaucomatous change in glaucoma suspects. Am J Ophthalmol 142:576–582

Li H K 1999 Telemedicine and ophthalmology. Surv Ophthalmol 44:61–72

Lim J I, LaBree L, Nichols T, Cardena I 2000 Fundus imaging with standard 35-millimeter slides for diabetic retinopathy. Ophthalmology 107:866–870

Lin A, Stern G 1998 Correlation between pterygium size and induced corneal astigmatism. Cornea 17:28–30

Lin D Y, Blumenkranz M S, Brothers R J, et al 2002 The sensitivity and specificity of single-field nonmydriatic monochromatic digital fundus photography with remote image interpretation for diabetic retinopathy screening: A comparison with ophthalmoscopy and standardised mydriatic color photography. Am J Ophthalmol 134:204–213

Liu Z, Huang A J, Pflugfelder S C 1999 Evaluation of corneal thickness and topography in normal eyes using the Orbscan corneal topography system. Br J Ophthalmol 83:774–778

McLaren J W, Brubaker R F 1983 Light sources for fluorescein fluorophotometry. Appl Opt 22:2897–2905

McMahon T T, Anderson R J, Roberts C, et al 2005 Repeatability of corneal topography measurement in keratoconus with the TMS-1. Optom Vis Sci 82:405–415

Macri A, Rolando M, Pflugfelder S 2000 A standardized visual scale for evaluation of tear fluorescein clearance. Ophthalmology 107:1338–1343

Manning F J, Wehrly S R, Foulks G N 1995 Patient tolerance and ocular surface staining characteristics of lissamine green versus rose bengal. Ophthalmology 102:1953–1957

Margrain T H, Boulton M, Marshall J, Sliney D H 2004 Do blue light filters confer protection against age-related macular degeneration? Prog Ret Eye Res 23:523–531

Mattern J, Mayer P R 1990 Excretion of fluorescein into breast milk [letter]. Am J Ophthalmol 109:598

Medeiros F A, Zangwill L M, Bowd C, Weinreb R N 2004 Comparison of the GDx VCC scanning laser polarimeter, HRT II confocal scanning laser ophthalmoscope, and stratus OCT optical coherence tomograph for the detection of glaucoma. Arch Ophthalmol 122:827–837

Mejia-Barbosa Y, Malacara-Hernandez D 2001 A review of methods for measuring corneal topography. Optom Vis Sci 87:240–253

Mengher L S, Bron A J, Tonge S R, Gilbert D J 1985 Effect of fluorescein instillation on the pre-corneal tear film stability. Curr Eye Res 4:9–12

Meyler J, Burnett Hodd N 1998 The use of digital image capture in contact lens practice. Contact Lens Anterior Eye 21:3–11

Moller-Pedersen T, Vogel M, Li H F, et al 1997 Quantification of stromal thinning, epithelial thickness, and corneal haze after photorefractive keratectomy using in vivo confocal microscopy. Ophthalmology 104:360–368

Morgan A J, Harper J, Hosking S L, Gilmartin B 2002 The effect of corneal thickness and corneal curvature on pneumatonometer measurements. Curr Eye Res 25:107–112

Newsom R S, Clover A, Costen M T, et al 2001 Effect of digital image compression on screening for diabetic retinopathy. Br J Ophthalmol 85:799–802

Norn M S 1973 Lissamine green – vital staining of cornea and conjunctiva. Acta Ophthalmol 51:483–491

Norn M S 1988 Tear fluid pH in normals, contact lens wearers, and pathological cases. Acta Ophthalmol 66:485–489

Novotny H R, Alvis D L 1961 A method of photographing fluorescent circulating blood in the human retina. Circulation 24:82–86

O'Donnell C, Wolffsohn J S 2004 Grading of corneal transparency. Contact Lens Anterior Eye 27:161–170

Owen C G 2000 Digital imaging in diabetic retinopathy. In: Rudnicka A R, Birch J (eds) Diabetic Eye Disease: Identification and Co-management. Butterworth-Heinemann, Oxford, p 107–112

Owen C G, Ellis T J, Rudnicka A R, Woodward E G 2002 Optimal green (red-free) digital imaging of conjunctival vasculature. Ophthalmic Physiol Opt 22:234–243

Papas E B 2000 Key factors in the subjective and objective assessment of conjunctival erythema. Invest Ophthalmol Vis Sci 41:687–691

Parikh R S, Parikh S R, Sekhar G C, et al 2007 Normal age-related decay of retinal nerve fiber layer thickness. Ophthalmology 114:921–926

Pavline C J, Sherar M D, Foster F S 1990 Subsurface ultrasound microscopic imaging of the intact eye. Ophthalmology 97:244–250

Pavline C J, Harasiewicz K, Foster F S 1992 Ultrasound biomicroscopy of anterior segment structures in normal and glaucomatous eyes. Am J Ophthalmol 113:381–389

Peterson R C, Wolffsohn J S 2005 The effect of digital image resolution and compression on anterior eye imaging. Br J Ophthalmol 89:828–830

Peterson R C, Wolffsohn J S, Fowler, C 2006 Optimization of anterior eye fluorescein viewing. Am J Ophthalmol 142:572–575

Pieroni C G, Witkin A J, Ko T H, et al 2006 Ultrahigh resolution optical coherence tomography in non-exudative age related macular degeneration. Br J Ophthalmol 90:191–197

Polito A, Del Borrello M, Polini G, et al 2006 Diurnal variation in clinically significant diabetic macular edema measured by the stratus OCT. Retina 26:14–20

Polunin G S, Kourenkov V V, Polunina E G 1998 Corneal transparency and measurement of corneal permeability in excimer laser photorefractive keratectomy. J Refract Surg 14:230–234

Popper M, Morgado A M, Quadrado M J, Van Best J A 2004 Corneal cell density measurement in vivo by scanning slit confocal microscopy: method and validation. Ophthalmic Res 36:270–276

Pugh J A, Van Jacobson J M, Heuven W A, et al 1993 Screening for diabetic retinopathy. The wide-angle retinal camera. Diabetes Care 16:889–895

Quigley H A, Addicks E M, Green W R 1982 Optic nerve damage in human glaucoma. III. Quantitative correlation of nerve fiber loss and visual field defect in glaucoma, ischemic neuropathy, papilledema, and toxic neuropathy. Arch Ophthalmol 100:135–146

Razvi F M, Kritzinger E E, Tsaloumas M D, Ryder R E J 2001 Use of oral fluorescein angiography in the diagnosis of macular oedema within a diabetic retinopathy screening programme. Diabet Med 18:1003

Reiser B J, Ignacio T S, Wang Y M, et al 2005 In vitro measurement of rabbit corneal epithelial thickness using ultrahigh resolution optical coherence tomography. Vet Ophthalmol 8:85–88

Reus N J, Lemij H G 2004a Diagnostic accuracy of the GDx VCC for glaucoma. Ophthalmology 111:1860–1865

Reus N J, Lemij H G 2004b The relationship between standard automated perimetry and GDx VCC measurements. Invest Ophthalmol Vis Sci 45:840–845

Rohrschneider K, Burk R O W, Kruse F E, Völcker H E 1994 Reproducibility of optic nerve head topography with a new laser tomographic scanning device. Ophthalmology 101:1044–1049

Romanchuk KG 1982 Fluorescein. Physiochemical factors affecting its fluorescence. Surv Ophthalmol 26:269–283

Roorda A, Zhang Y H, Duncan J L 2007 High-resolution in vivo imaging of the RPE mosaic in eyes with retinal disease. Invest Opthalmol Vis Sci 48:2297–2303

Rudnicka A R, Burk R O W, Edgar D F, Fitzke F W 1998 Magnification characteristics of fundus imaging systems. Ophthalmology 105:2186–2192

Rudnisky C J, Hinz B J, de Tennant M T, et al 2002 High-resolution stereoscopic digital fundus photography versus contact lens biomicroscopy for the detection of clinically significant macular edema. Ophthalmology 109:267–274

Ruggeri M, Webbe H, Jiao S L, et al 2007 In vivo three-dimensional high-resolution imaging of rodent retina with spectral-domain optical coherence tomography. Invest Ophthalmol Vis Sci. 48:1808–1814

Ryder R J, Kong N, Bates A S, et al 1998 Instant electronic imaging systems are superior to Polaroid at detecting sight threatening diabetic retinopathy. Diabet Med 15:254–258

Sa H S, Kyung S E, Oh S Y 2005 Extraocular muscle imaging in complex strabismus. Ophthalmic Surg Lasers Imag 36:487–493

Santodomingo-Rubido J, Mallen E A H, Gilmartin B, Wolffsohn J S 2002 A new non-contact optical device for ocular biometry. Br J Ophthalmol 86:458–462

Schirmer K E 2004 Digital photos through the microscope's oculars. Rev Ophthalmol 11:59–62

Shiba T, Maruo K, Akahoshi T 1999 Development of a multi-field fundus photographing system using a non-mydriatic camera for diabetic retinopathy. Diabetes Res Clin Pract 45:1–8

Singh K D, Logan N S, Gilmartin B 2006 Three-dimensional modelling of the human eye based on magnetic resonance imaging. Invest Ophthalmol Vis Sci 47:2272–2279

Sinthanayothin C, Boyce J, Cook H, et al 1999 Automated localisation of the optic disc, fovea, and retinal blood vessels from digital colour fundus images. Br J Ophthalmol 83:902–910

Smith G T, Brown N A, Shun-Shin G A 1990 Light scatter from the central human cornea. Eye 4:584–588

Soya K, Amano S, Oshika T 2002 Quantification of simulated corneal haze by measuring back-scattered light. Ophthalmic Res 34:380–388

Swindale N V, Stjepanovic G, Chin A, Mikelberg F S 2000 Automated analysis of normal and glaucomatous optic nerve head topography images. Invest Ophthalmol Vis Sci 41:1730–1742

Tabery H M 2003 Corneal surface changes in keratoconjunctivitis sicca. Part I: The surface proper. A non-contact photomicrographic in vivo study in the human cornea. Eye 17:482–487

Tan J C H, Hitchings R A 2003 Approach for identifying glaucomatous optic nerve progression by scanning laser tomography. Invest Ophthalmol Vis Sci 44:2621–2626

Technical Advisory Service for Images (TASi) 2003 Advice paper on digital cameras. June, 1–21. Online. Available: http://www.tasi.ac.uk

Tervo T, Moilanen J 2003 In vivo confocal microscopy for evaluation of wound healing following corneal refractive surgery. Prog Ret Eye Res 22:339–358

Torens S, Berger E, Stave J, Guthoff R 2000 Laser scanning microscopy for imaging the microarchitecture and dynamics of break-up phenomena of the preocular tear film. Ophthalmologe 97:635–639

Tuulonen A, Ohinmaa T, Alanko H I, et al 1999 The application of teleophthalmology in examining patients with glaucoma: a pilot study. J Glaucoma 8:367–373

Urbak S F 1998 Ultrasound biomicroscopy. I. Precision of measurements. Acta Ophthalmol Scand 76:447–455

Urbak S F 1999 Ultrasound biomicroscopy. III. Accuracy and agreement of measurements. Acta Ophthalmol Scand 77:293–297

Urbak S F, Pedersen J K, Thorsen T T 1998 Ultrasound biomicroscopy. II. Intraobserver and interobserver reproducibility of measurements. Acta Ophthalmol Scand 76:546–549

van de Pol C, Soya K, Hwang D G 2001 Objective assessment of transient corneal haze and its relation to visual performance after photorefractive keratectomy. Am J Ophthalmol 132:204–210

Wang J, Fonn D, Simpson T L, Jones L 2003 Precorneal and pre- and postlens tear film thickness measured indirectly with optical coherence tomography. Invest Ophthalmol Vis Sci 44:2524–2528

Wang L, Gaigalas A K 2002 Quantitating fluorescence intensity from fluorophores: practical use of MESF values. J Res Natl Inst Stand Technol 107:339–353

Watson A P, Rosen E S 1990 Oral fluorescein angiography: reassessment of its relative safety and evaluation of optimum conditions with use of capsules. Br J Ophthalmol 74:458–461

Wegener A, Laser H 2001 Image-analysis and Scheimpflug-photography in the anterior segment of the eye – a review article. Klin Monatsbl Augenheilkd 218:67–77

Weinberger D, Stiebel-Kalish H, Priel E, et al 1999 Digital red free photography for the evaluation of retinal blood vessel displacement in epiretinal membranes. Ophthalmology 106:1380–1383

Whited J D 2006 Accuracy and reliability of teleophthalmology for diagnosing diabetic retinopathy and macular edema: A review of the literature. Diabetes Technol Therapeut 8:102–111

Wolffsohn J S 2004 Incremental nature of anterior eye grading scales determined by objective image analysis. Br J Ophthalmol 88:1434–1438

Wolffsohn J S, Peterson R C 2006 Anterior ophthalmic imaging. Clin Exp Optom 89:205–214

Wolffsohn J S, Purslow C 2003 Clinical monitoring of ocular physiology using digital image analysis. Contact Lens Anterior Eye 26:27–35

Wollstein G, Garway-Heath D F, Hitchings R A 1998 Identification of early glaucoma cases with the scanning laser ophthalmoscope. Ophthalmology 105:1557–1563

Wollstein G, Garway-Heath D F, Fontana L, Hitchings R A 2000 Identifying early glaucomatous changes: Comparison between expert clinical assessment of optic disc photographs and confocal scanning ophthalmoscopy. Ophthalmology 107:2272–2277

Yasuno Y, Madjarova V D, Makita S, et al 2005 Three-dimensional and high-speed swept-source optical coherence tomography for in vivo investigation of human anterior eye segments. Opt Express 13:10652–10664

Yogesan K, Constable I J, Eikelboom R H, van Saarloos P P 1998 Tele-ophthalmic screening using digital imaging devices. Aust NZ J Ophthalmol 26:9–11

Zangwill L M, Weinreb R N, Berry C C, et al 2004 The confocal scanning laser ophthalmoscopy ancillary study to the ocular hypertension treatment study: Study design and baseline factors. Am J Ophthalmol 137:219–227

Zantos S G 1983 Cystic formations in the corneal epithelium during extended wear of contact lenses. Int Contact Lens Clin 10:128–168

Zhou Q, Weinreb R N 2002 Individualized compensation of anterior segment birefringence during scanning laser polarimetry. Invest Ophthalmol Vis Sci 43:2221–2228

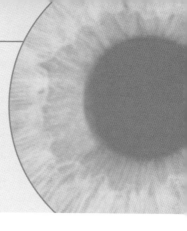

Subject Index